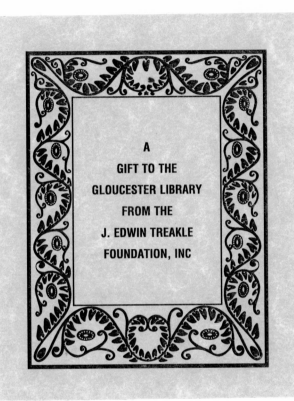

EMT Rescue

Pat Ivey

AN [e-*reads*]BOOK
New York, NY

Copyright © 1993 by Pat Ivey
First e-reads publication 2002
www.e-reads.com
ISBN 0-7592-4464-2

EMT: BEYOND THE LIGHTS AND SIRENS was dedicated to my children, David, Matt and Jennifer, for bringing light and joy to my life.

EMT: RESCUE is dedicated to my parents, Edna and Al Follmar, for teaching me that love was meant to be shared.

And to the memory of Mary Kay Mayo
1980-1992

I was a stranger, and ye took me in:
Naked, and ye clothed me: I was sick, and ye visited me:
I was in prison, and ye came unto me.
MATTHEW 25: 35-36

LAKE OF THE WOODS VOLUNTEER RESCUE SQUAD 1993

Purvis Beanum

Mike Beery

Pia Boot

Holly Brim

Joe Broderick

Mara Bueng

Phyllis Burbank

Bill Carter

Kirk Clayberg

Rachel Coon

Kathy Davis

Maurice Dionne

Phil Dorn

Norm Ensrud

Wes Eubanks

Judy Gill

Sally Goodrich

Art Gourdier

Ken Haase

Jan Haase

Ed Hill

Pat Ivey

Kathryn Janeski

Mac Johnson

Debbie Katcher

Jack Kelley

Christie Kelley

Bobby Lane

Paul Lewis

Tracey Luebkert

Jack LeMay

Becky Naca

Donna Oliver

Scott Parkinson

Andy Powers

Tom Reeder

Barbara Robinson

Doris Smith

Dick Smith

Bill Werber

Darren Zunno

Jerady Zunno

Table of Contents

Prologue

On the Kindness of Strangers

EMT: Beyond the Lights and Sirens began as a journal, a personal account of my experiences on my community volunteer rescue squad, tracing my steps, slow and often unsteady, into the world of emergency prehospital medicine.

I have heard and continue to hear from Emergency Medical Technicians throughout the world. Bill Trumbore from Effort, Pennsylvania, wrote in his letter to me: "While reading your book I laughed and cried with you. I came to realize that what we do and what we feel is universal to those of us who endeavor in our line of work."

He is right. For we have all been on the same roads, dirt and gravel and paved. We have knelt over the same patients in the same rooms, cramped and hot from corner wood-stoves. We have held children in our arms and in our hearts and heard the cries of families, heart-wrenching cries that mingle with our own silent ones. And our prayers are the same, in whatever language.

I have heard from men and women from Poultney, Vermont, and La Grange Park, Illinois; from Ashburnham, Maine, and Port Charlotte and Bradenton, Florida; Gullford, Connecticut, and Kenmore, New York; from Shreveport, Louisiana, and Nebraska City, Nebraska; from Billings, Montana, and Renfrewshire, Scotland, and a tiny village in Portugal.

I've heard from teenagers who've discovered *Beyond the Lights and Sirens* in their school libraries and decided to become junior members of their community rescue squads, and I've heard from families who've been touched by the skill and kindness of volunteer rescue squad personnel.

"You reminded me why I became an EMT," wrote Tim Dodson of New Orleans, Louisiana. Paul and JoAnn Best from Waldo, Arkansas, shared with me stories of their rural volunteer squad. Despite his hearing disability, Robert Drake, a student at Gallaudet University, wants so very much to be an EMT. I have heard from so many who say to me, "If you could do it, so can I!" And, of course, they can.

I've heard from people who just want to talk, to share the stories of their "saves" and their losses. Mike, an EMT from Ohio, called me one rainy day. "It's raining here, too," he said. Then he told me that one of my dreams had become a reality for him: he had delivered a baby. His words were without the exhilaration I expected. He was quiet for several moments. "We had another call there," he said, finally. "SIDS (Sudden Infant Death Syndrome)" he told me, grief still resounding in his voice, " — the baby I'd delivered was dead."

I have been asked, "Do you still have Jesse's sock?"

I do.

It's in the same dresser drawer.

It's a reminder of that cool October morning when we struggled to save his life.

That small red sock continues to remind me of why we are here, why we endure the battle even when the odds are so overwhelming.

It is a reminder of hope that is eternal, of memories that sustain and strengthen us, and of love that makes it all complete . . . a reminder of what we take with us and what we bestow within and beyond our world of lights and sirens.

One

"Possible Overdose," The dispatcher said. "Thirty-four-year-old female."

The location of the call was near my house. Otherwise, I might not have gone. Kirk and Bobby and Pia were on duty and easily could have handled it.

I pulled my uniform from the closet and slipped it on over my shorts, grabbed my portable radio, and headed for the car. "Possible overdose" doesn't tell us much. It doesn't tell us what was taken, or the level of consciousness, or the respiratory status. Deputies often accompany us to overdose calls for adults because of the likelihood of a volatile situation. With children, the overdose is almost always accidental; with adults, it's intentional.

Our security force was already on the scene. Clay met me at the driveway.

"I don't think she's taken anything, Pat," he said, shaking his head. "Her neighbor called us and then called for rescue. He said she was acting funny, but this isn't the first time."

"What's she doing?" I asked him.

"Reading from the Bible. Saying she's got to get rid of the devil. She needs some help, Pat, but I don't think she's taken any pills. We've been here before, just to ask her to quiet down."

"What's her name?"

"Lisa Wilkins."

I heard the siren in the distance and reached for my radio. "EMS 29 to Medic 292."

"Go ahead, EMS 29," Bobby responded.

"Come in easy," I told him.

3

On the front porch, a small boy played quietly with plastic toy dinosaurs.

"Hi," I said, kneeling beside him. "My name is Pat. An ambulance will be here in a minute just to make sure your Mommy's okay."

He nodded slowly and held a dinosaur up for me to see. "I'm Tyler and this is a Tyrannosaurus rex," he said.

"The king of all the dinosaurs," I replied.

He smiled then, but only with his mouth. There was no sparkle in his eyes. There was no luster in his pale, slender face.

His mother was standing in the kitchen reading aloud from her Bible. Her back was to me, and I approached her quietly. "Lisa," I said, but she seemed unaware of my presence until I reached out and touched her arm. She wore a sleeveless shirt, and her skin was cool to the touch. She turned and looked at me, her dark eyes dazed and vacant.

"And the children of Israel again did evil in the sight of the Lord." Her finger moved slowly, deliberately across the lines. "Listen!" she said, and she read it to me again.

"Lisa," I began, "we want to know that you are all right." My words sounded hollow, even to me, for it was quite clear she was not. "We would like to take you to see the doctor."

"I am not sick," she said. "I am evil."

"I don't think you are evil," I responded. "Sometimes things get very confusing for us. Sometimes life is very difficult — "

"I am evil and I want to speak to a minister," she interrupted me. "This book says I'm evil. The Bible says I'm evil. I don't need you. I want to speak to a minister."

"All right," I told her.

We summoned the local minister. Bobby and Kirk stayed on the porch with Tyler and played dinosaur games. Lisa was eager to sign the refusal form, which stated that she did not want us to treat or transport her. We were not so eager to leave. Kirk and Bobby lifted Tyler to the ambulance. He listened to his own heartbeat with the stethoscope and put a Snoopy Band-Aid on an imaginary cut. Kirk gave him a small stuffed dragon to go with his dinosaur collection.

Pia and I stayed close to Lisa while we waited for the minister to arrive. She would not leave the kitchen, and continued to read to us from the Bible. We pulled chairs in from the dining room and sat in a circle next to the sink, where dishes were piled high. Lisa showed us a scar on her arm where she'd once had a tattoo, then had it burned away. "It was Satan," she said.

When the minister arrived, Clay was the first to leave, having determined that the scene was secure. Lisa and the minister sat together, still in the kitchen. I placed my hand on her shoulder before Pia and I left, but she was again unaware of my presence. Her head was lowered over the Bible, her dark, unkempt hair obscuring her face.

"Please call if you need us," I said softly to the minister. He nodded.

Kirk flashed the lights of the ambulance for Tyler as they drove away. The small boy watched them from the porch, his hand half raised in farewell. I drove the short distance back to my house.

It was not quite nine o'clock on that beautiful May morning in 1992. My older son, David, would be home from Austin the next day. His year in VISTA was over, and he was coming home for three months before leaving for Ecuador and two years of service in the Peace Corps. Matt, finishing his first year at the University of Arkansas in Fayetteville, would be home by the weekend. There was much to do.

I thought of Lisa and Tyler many times throughout the morning. I hadn't learned much about her from Clay. I did know she was a single parent, trying to raise her child by herself. She'd recently lost her job and was growing more and more isolated.

My children and I had made it through separation and divorce. It had not been easy, and it had surely taken its toll, but we had survived. Why is it, I wondered, that some of us survive and others don't? And when is it that we lose the ability to cope; when do misfortune and heartbreak take on the shape, the silhouette of demons, and at what point do hallucinations become real and fill not only the corners of our minds, but also, finally, the corners of our rooms?

I drove into Fredericksburg that afternoon to do some last minute shopping. Ingredients for lasagna and banana nut bread were high on my list. Jennifer and I would fix her brothers' favorites. She was fifteen then — sometimes we giggled together over silly things and hugged each other tightly; other times, we both struggled with her quest for independence.

It was three-thirty when I turned into Lake of the Woods, my home now for sixteen years. On my right was our Volunteer Rescue Squad and Fire Department. I stopped briefly to get my mail and to look over the call sheets to see if there had been any emergencies while I was in town. Nothing since the call for Lisa.

Jennifer's bus went by as I left the building. I picked her up at the next stop. "Hi," she said to me. "Why did you pick me up here?"

"Just so I'd get to spend more time with you," I told her.

"Can I switch the radio station?" Her hand was on the dial before I answered, and Garth Brooks was suddenly transformed to the Red Hot Chili Peppers.

Just as we turned onto Yorktown, our street, the tones went off. "Attention Lake of the Woods Rescue Squad, unresponsive child on Lakeview Drive. Expedite."

I knew it was Tyler.

". . . because Erica said she was going to the dance with Robert and Robert said he didn't know what she was talking about — "

"Jennifer," I interrupted her.

"I hate it when you say my name that way," she sighed. "I always think I'm in trouble."

"Rescue 292 is en route to the scene." It was Kirk. "Additional personnel respond to the scene." His voice, usually strong and self-assured was shaky. He, too, knew it was Tyler.

"No," I assured her. "You're not in trouble. Get your things together. I'm going to drop you off at the house. I've got to go on this call."

Lisa had thanked the minister for taking the time to talk with her. Yes, she assured him, she was fine. Talking was all she had needed. She walked him to the door and out onto the porch. She reached down and mussed Tyler's hair, a loving gesture, waved good-bye to the minister, and retreated into the house.

When Tyler got hungry for lunch he left the porch and went into the kitchen. He moved the chair to the counter and climbed on it to reach the peanut butter. He moved quietly, sidestepping his mother, who stood in the kitchen holding the open Bible, reading softly to herself. He ate his sandwich on the front porch, then carried the dinosaurs and stuffed dragon into the front yard. The Tyrannosaurus rex and

Brontosaurus peeked out above the fresh May grass. Tyler hummed a happy tune from *Sesame Street*.

She told him they were going for a swim. He stood up and reached for her hand and they walked the short distance to the lake, to the water's edge. He carried the small green stuffed dragon in his free hand; in hers, she carried her leatherbound Bible.

On the lakeside road, a front seat passenger was the first to notice the woman and boy in the water. She commented to her husband, "It's awfully cool for swimming, don't you think?" He readily agreed, but neither of them noticed that the woman and the boy were fully clothed.

The driver of the second car to pass thought the two were playing in the water. He slowed down for a closer look, then sped away to report what he'd seen; but by the time he reached the security office, two other people had called to report a woman in the lake attempting to drown a child.

Tyler broke free. He was almost home when he tripped and fell. A neighbor had heard his screams and rushed to him, arriving just as he lost consciousness: terrified and winded from the struggle and the long run home, he had fainted.

When I arrived at the house, I found Tyler bundled in a blanket, awake and responsive, in the neighbor's arms. "I lost my dragon," he said. His voice cracked as he spoke. "He drowned in the water," he told me, and he began to cry. The neighbor held him tightly.

"I'll get you another one, Tyler, just as soon as the ambulance gets here. You can have your pick," I said, reaching for his small, pale hand.

When security reached the site of the reported drowning, Lisa was standing waist-deep in the water.

"Satan is here," she screamed at them. "Let me baptize you before Satan lays his hands on you."

They got in the water with her. She didn't resist them when they picked her up and carried her to the car. They brought her to us, her Bible clutched tightly in her hand, and we lifted her onto the ambulance. She shivered as Pia and I removed her clothes and covered her with blankets.

"Read to me," she said, finally relinquishing the Bible and handing it to me.

"In a moment, Lisa," I responded. "I will in just a moment."

While we took her pulse and blood pressure, Kirk carried a teddy bear and a stuffed brown rabbit with floppy ears to Tyler. Joe was there with him. He, too, had driven to the scene, and was helping Al and his wife with Tyler. Although Tyler seemed fine except for a scraped knee, they had talked to the doctor and were planning to take him for a checkup. Joe told him we were taking his mother to see the doctor, too.

"Will she be all right?" he asked. "Will Mommy come back home?"

When we answer such a question, we hope that our response will not be a lie, that there will be some truth in it, especially when the question comes from a child. "Yes, she'll be all right," Joe answered. "And she'll come home as soon as she can."

When we pulled away, Tyler waved.

"Don't use the siren until we get out on Route 3," I told Kirk. "And only when it's necessary," I added. I was concerned that it would only alarm Tyler. Lisa might also be startled by the sudden wail.

Lisa continued to tremble, and Pia tucked more blankets around her. I reached for the Bible. The pages were wet and difficult to pry apart. Her eyes were fixed on me. I turned to the book of Matthew, and read:

Blessed are the poor in spirit: for theirs is the kingdom of heaven. Blessed are they that mourn: for they shall be comforted. Blessed are the meek: for they shall inherit the earth. Blessed are they which do hunger and thirst after righteousness: for they shall be filled. Blessed are the merciful: for they shall obtain mercy. Blessed are the pure in heart: for they shall see God.

She closed her eyes and was quiet en route to Culpeper Memorial Hospital, but she was not at peace. Her body never relaxed. The shivering never stopped. When we arrived, we moved her gently from the gurney onto the stretcher. "I don't know you," she said, her eyes wide and apprehensive. "But I love you."

"We love you, too, Lisa," I told her.

That evening a sheriff's deputy drove her to Western State Hospital in Staunton, a Virginia facility for patients with psychological problems. Tyler's father came to get his son.

And that night I listened to the rest of the story of Erica and Robert while Jennifer and I made the sauce for the lasagna and baked two loaves of banana nut bread.

Two

It was in October 1981 that I began my journey into the world of emergency medicine. My first steps were unsure, and I carried with me uncertainties rooted in fear and ignorance.

Nineteen eighty-one was the year the first test-tube baby was born in the United States. That year, the price of stamps rose to twenty cents, and Sandra Day O'Connor was the first woman appointed to the Supreme Court. In October 1981, Ronald Reagan was in the tenth month of his presidency. That same month, I submitted my application to the Lake of the Woods Rescue Squad.

The world has turned many times since that month, that year. Many seasons have passed. Enhanced 911 has come to Orange County, and many of the dirt and gravel roads we traveled are now paved. We have lost our first patient to gunshot wounds in a drug deal gone sour, a seventeen-year-old boy shot at point-blank range on a dark country road.

Late at night, I hear the cows mooing from a nearby meadow. My house sits in the flight pattern of the Canada geese. My ears are attuned to their honking, and when I hear them in the distance, I move quickly from whatever I am doing so I can run outside to my deck and watch them in their perfect V above me.

We are a rural rescue squad. There are thirty-seven of us, and we are all volunteers. As an EMT/CPR Instructor, I have taught thirty-one of them, and now I am their Captain. I tell them they are like my children to me. They are good and dedicated people, and it is my job to take care of them.

It was a springlike October day. She was helping her husband. Something was wrong with the drive shaft, he'd told her. They lay beneath the truck, inspecting it. Then he eased out from under the truck and climbed into the driver's seat.

"I'll start it," he called to her. It would be easier to see the problem. He turned the key, and the heavy engine bellowed. As he stepped from the truck, it slipped into gear.

We were on duty that day, Joe and Dick and I. We had been dispatched to Orange, twenty-five miles away, for a possible heart attack. Our patient was an eighty-eight-year-old man who'd had eight heart attacks in three years. His chief complaint on that day was weakness and dizziness. In a healthy person those symptoms might not be serious, but with this man's medical history, weakness and dizziness could be the prelude to cardiac arrest. We put him on high-flow oxygen and I started an IV.

We were on our way to Martha Jefferson Hospital in Charlottesville when we heard snatches of conversation on the radio: ". . . injury . . . Spotsylvania County . . . 293 . . ." The transmission was broken and heavy with static, but we recognized Norm's voice.

"Another call," I remarked to Joe. "Injury."

He acknowledged me, nodding. "Pulse is still 84 and strong," he said.

I leaned forward. "No chest pain or tightness?" I asked our patient. I reached for his hand as he shook his head, no. It was cool but dry, and that was good: diaphoresis, heavy perspiration, is another warning sign. "And no difficulty breathing?" Again, he shook his head. "Good," I said to him, "We'll be there in about ten minutes."

We are lucky; we have regularly scheduled duty crews. This was our day to serve. But we were forty miles away when the tones went off for the second call.

Norm was the first one to arrive, then Mike and Scott, just back from class. Kathy, heading home from work, had reached the building just as they were about to leave, and had asked if she could go.

"It's an injury," Norm had called to her. "Probably nothing serious but come on," he said, waving.

The deputy on the scene called it a terrible tragedy. When the truck had slipped into gear, it had rolled over the woman. She'd screamed once, no more; it was too difficult to draw a breath.

Their neighbor, hearing the scream, called 911. "A woman's hurt," she said. And gave no more information.

11

The victim was free of the truck when they arrived on the scene. Her husband was frantic. Norm tried to get the woman onto the backboard. Mike tried to hold oxygen on her, but she fought him. Her legs were crushed. Her abdomen was split open. She tore the oxygen off and attempted to sit up, but her ribs and sternum were in fragments and had sliced open her lungs, and sitting up would not help. They carried her to the ambulance and placed her on the gurney and marked en route to Mary Washington Hospital, asking for a medic unit to meet them en route.

"For morphine," Norm told me. "There was nothing else we could do." Within a mile of her house, she died.

They took her to the morgue. Then Norm called Leroy Gardner, the director of our emergency medical services council and a member of the local Critical Incident Stress Debriefing Team. Leroy hurried to the hospital and talked with them, telling them what they might expect: perhaps sleeplessness that night; and there could be nightmares. And it's all right to cry, he told them.

"My worst calls," Kirk tells me, "are the calls where we weren't expecting how bad it would be. We're not really prepared," be says. "Like we've been told it's a call for 'chest pains' and we get on the scene and find it's cardiac arrest."

And I think of Norm and Scott and Kathy and Mike and the call for "an injury."

Kirk graduated from the University of Virginia with a major in biology and a minor in psychology, then went on to Virginia Commonwealth University, and is working toward a degree in forensics. He joined the squad in February 1991. He is twenty-four years old, a quiet, pensive young man, slender and of medium height, with sharp, angular features.

"The trailer fire," he said, his eyes, deep-set and hazel, meeting mine.

Jack and Sally and Norm had been on duty. Kirk was covering for Pia. It was a brisk and windy fall afternoon, and when they arrived on the scene, the entire area was dark with smoke. They set up the aid station away from the fire, but close enough to assist the firefighters. They carried the trauma box and oxygen from the ambulance and placed them on the tarp they'd spread on the ground. Next, they got the water and cups. Sally smiled at Kirk. "All set."

Luther, one of our five then, found the man at the rear of the trailer. It appeared he'd sought safety in the bedroom, and then when the fire spread — and with barns and trailers, fire spreads quickly — he hadn't had a chance. Luther picked up the man, still in a crouching position, still smoldering, and carried him outside.

"We've got a patient over here," Luther called, and laid him down on the ground.

Kirk and Sally rushed toward him. They knelt on either side. Sally touched him, then quickly withdrew her hand. His body was hot and dry and hard, his arm set at a ninety-degree angle. Luther had said they had a patient, and Kirk and Sally, so new to the squad, thought that the victim needed care. Sally reached in her pocket for a face mask. Kirk removed the remaining fragments of the man's shirt.

Ray Harvey, cardiac technician for Battlefield Rescue and a neighbor of this man, approached them. He put his hand on Sally's back. "He's gone," he said softly. "Nothing can be done now."

I called the Critical Incident Stress Debriefing Team from Fredericksburg to meet with Sally and Kirk and Luther and others who were there that day. "Most of the people at the debriefing said it didn't really affect them that badly," Kirk told me. "Sally and I, I think, seemed to be the ones most upset by it. But — ," he shrugged, " — sometimes it's hard to tell."

A year later, and out of the blue, he said to me, "Whenever I clean the chimney in my house, I remember. The smell . . . the smell brings me back."

It was just past dawn on a hot and humid July morning. The tones jolted me from deep sleep. The dispatcher announced "chest pains," and I tried to think of who was on duty for the day. Kirk and Art, I remembered, and Bill for advanced life support. It was a lazy Saturday morning, and sleeping in felt good.

He was only forty. He'd been complaining of some vague chest tightness for over a week. He'd even gone to the doctor, but after waiting for fifteen minutes in the downtown office, being an impatient man, he'd walked out. The pains awakened him. His wife was already up, and when she heard him in the bathroom she put the bacon in the frying pan.

The children, three girls and a boy, awoke to the sweet smell and gathered in the kitchen. After breakfast, instead of remaining at the table to smoke, he moved into the living room so he could stretch out on the sofa.

"Indigestion," he complained to his wife, rubbing his chest.

"I'll bring you some soda," she answered.

When he lay down, the pain worsened, and as she walked into the living room, she was shocked by his face, suddenly pale and wet with perspiration. She took his hand. It felt cold and clammy.

"Help me sit up," he told her. "I can't seem to get my breath."

They had no phone, but they lived within walking distance of the security building and the dispatcher. The oldest daughter ran there. "My father's having chest pains," she cried. Bob tried to get the information from her, but as soon as she gave the address, she turned and was gone.

Art was first to the building. Then Kirk. Bill lived further away. "We'll be en route momentarily," Kirk announced.

In my room, lying sleepily in my bed, I heard him. His voice was strong, assured.

"Directions, please," he asked.

"Take a left onto Route 3," Mike began.

"Wait — " Kirk interrupted him.

No pen, I thought to myself. We all do it. We ask for directions, then realize we've stuck the pen in our pocket.

The girl had rushed back home. She heard the crying before she entered the house. Her younger sister yelled, "He's not breathing. He's dead." Her mother was leaning over him, trying to blow air into his mouth. The son, very young and frightened, was sitting on the floor, crying.

"Where are they?" she called to her daughter. "Didn't you get the rescue squad?"

Again, the daughter ran, this time to the rescue building. She saw the lights of the ambulance and rushed toward it as Kirk was asking for directions. "Mama says he's dead," she cried. "Hurry!" She climbed into the back of the ambulance. "Come on. I'll show you where we live."

"Cardiac arrest," Kirk said into the radio, and his voice was shaky and sorrowful.

I moved quickly from my bed.

"We're en route," Kirk told the dispatcher. "Additional personnel meet us on the scene."

Kirk and Art had been EMTs for just over a month. This was their first code. They pulled onto Route 3. Bill was behind them now. They headed west and turned down a narrow road that dwindled into nothing more than a trail. The ambulance shook, and in the back, the metal clipboard crashed onto the floor. The girl cried softly.

At the scene, Kirk rushed inside. Art grabbed the airways, oxygen, and bag mask. Bill stepped into the ambulance and retrieved the lifepack. Inside the house Kirk found the man on the floor, his wife over him struggling awkwardly, trying to do CPR.

She moved away when Kirk touched her shoulder, and he knelt, opened the airway, and checked for breathing. Properly done. By the book. *Determine breathlessness. Ventilate twice.* Kirk reached for his pocket mask. Phlegm and vomitus gurgled in the man's throat. Kirk turned aside momentarily, then turned back and ventilated twice. Barbara was soon beside him, and Art and Wes and Bill. I arrived next, then Joe and Jerady and Bobby.

We worked twenty minutes in the house, but it was dark and musty, and difficult to move. It took me two attempts to start the IV. Bobby inserted an EOA tube. The rhythm was ventricular fibrillation: the heart was only quivering, nothing more. We shocked three times, administered epinephrine and lidocaine in between. The monitor displayed straightline, asystole, no heartbeat.

Jerady was with the wife and children in the kitchen, and as we moved our patient from the house, I was aware of the family. In my memory, they sit huddled together, and I am reminded of a painting I have seen in the National Gallery of Art of women and children knotted together for protection against a raging storm.

Our struggle to resuscitate continued during the twenty-five minute trip to Mary Washington Hospital. We grew tired and took turns doing compressions. We'd used all our epinephrine. Barbara was behind us in her van, with the family. I glanced back at them from time to time and felt how awful it must be for them, not knowing . . . and at the same time, certain.

He was only forty years old, and so the resuscitation efforts were continued for another twenty minutes at the hospital before they finally pronounced him dead.

We were there for over an hour. We saw his wife and children before we left, still pressed tightly together. We spoke our condolences and offered assistance. If ever a family looked helpless and strong at the same time, it was this one.

We discussed the call on our way home.

"If he had just seen the doctor," Art said.

"Denial," Bill responded. "That's why over half of all AMI patients die outside the hospital. They wait and wait, swearing it must be a pulled muscle or indigestion or anything other than what it is."

"And then we get there and it's too late." Kirk's words were quiet and subdued. I detected a trace of anger.

"We did all we could," I said to him. And I thought of Lou and the baby we'd worked on years ago, four months old and dead in our arms. I put my hand on his shoulder. I didn't want to tell him it would get easier. It was not the time. Those words could come later.

But it does get easier. At least, sometimes I think it does.

On a cold March evening in 1989 we had a call for an accident on Route 3 at Lignum. There's a bad curve there. A young woman had lost control of her car and slammed into a telephone pole. She had deep facial lacerations and a compound fracture of the knee.

Paul and Rachel and I took care of her. Rachel got in the back seat to stabilize her head while I did a quick assessment and bandaged the lacerations. Paul helped me with the extrication device and with splinting her leg. We cut away most of her clothes during our assessment, then covered her with the blanket from our unit.

We were moving her onto the backboard slowly because even the slightest motion caused intense pain. I knew it had to be slow, but I was beginning to worry about the cold. Then, when they had her halfway out of the car, a woman stepped out of the crowd and came toward us with a blanket.

"Can you use this?" she asked me.

"Oh, yes," I told her. "Thank you. That's just what we need."

I tucked the blanket around our patient, and when I turned back, the woman was gone.

Several weeks later, she called me.

"I don't know if you remember me," she said. "I left my blanket with you at the wreck in Lignum. My name's Barbara Robinson. I was wondering if you still have my blanket."

"Sure, I remember you. You were the answer to my prayers that day," I told her. "It was freezing and we only had one blanket on the ambulance. We left your blanket at the hospital. I'm sure you can pick it up there."

"Was the woman all right?" she asked.

"She'll have to have some therapy for her knee, but she's going to be fine."

"That's good," she said, and I could hear the caring in her voice.

She told me she lived in Lignum and worked in Warrenton. She was the assistant superintendent of public works. "Sounds important, doesn't it?" she said, laughing. "I'm just in charge of street maintenance and snow removal and things like that."

"That's very important to me," I told her. "I don't do too well with anything frozen on the road."

"I heard your call on my scanner," she said, "and thought I might be able to help with traffic control. I've done that, too."

"Maybe you'd like to take an EMT class," I suggested to her. "I just started one."

She was quiet for a moment.

"No," she said, "not right now." But she gave me her address and phone number and asked me to let her know when I was going to teach the next class.

It was in October of the following year. I sent Barbara a card announcing the class. "I hope to see you on Thursday night," I wrote, then added, "I've kept the piece of paper with your name and address on it for a year and a half. This is very unusual for me so I think you are destined to be in this class."

And she was there.

Much later, she told me that the night she climbed the steps and walked into the classroom was the first time she'd done anything entirely on her own, without knowing anyone else. "I didn't even go to the hospital and get the blanket," she admitted. "I just went to Kmart and bought another one."

It's hard to believe that now.

Barbara is thirty-four years old and lives with her husband and daughter in a double-wide trailer on eighteen acres in Culpeper County, " — with my ducks and dogs and squirrels," she says. "I enjoy the solitude."

She is the natural daughter of an East German refugee and was adopted by her American parents while they were in the military and stationed in Germany. "I was twelve years old and couldn't speak any English," she told me. "I've come a long way."

We had a call in Spotsylvania County for a twenty-six-year-old woman who was "very weak and dizzy." Before we got to the scene, our dispatcher reported, "Patient has now left the residence."

We pulled up in front of the house and I got off the ambulance. "Barbara, you and Christie stay here with Joe," I said. "I'll just see what's going on."

The front porch was rotted away. I stepped across the moldy, splintered wood, and knocked on the screen door. I could see nothing but darkness.

"Just let the bitch go," a man yelled from inside.

I turned and walked back to the ambulance. "Joe, call for a deputy."

A woman approached us from the adjoining yard. "Don't pay no attention to him," she said. "That's her boyfriend. He won't do nothing. He's all mouth. She's been awful sick with high blood pressure, even fainted yesterday, but she won't go back to the doctor. I'm the one who called for you."

"Where did she go?" I asked.

"Behind the house, in the field," she said, gesturing toward the high grass at the back of the yard.

"She can't be far," Barbara said,

"She ain't," the woman agreed. "I find her myself all the time. Pretty little thing, don't know why she puts up with that bastard. That's what he is, you know, even if he is my brother."

"Okay, Barbara, get the portable radio and you and Christie check the field. We'll wait for the deputy."

"I'll go back inside and give him a piece of my mind," the woman said. "No woman ought to have to put up with that trash."

The deputy pulled into the drive as Barbara and Christie started across the field.

"The man's in the house," I told him. "He sounds threatening. I'm not sure what's going on here but I thought it would be good if you were around."

"Yeah," he said, nodding. "I've been here before. Guy gets plastered and then gets offensive. I've always thought he hits her but I can't get her to say anything."

"Portable 291 to Medic 291." It was Barbara.

"Go ahead, Portable 291," I responded.

"She's out here."

"We'll be right there," I told her.

"I'll stay and keep an eye on the house," the deputy said. "He's probably in there passed out."

Joe and I circled around behind the house until we saw Christie waving to us. We drove into the field from the road. When the girl spotted us, she got up and started to run.

"Stay there," Barbara told us over the portable.

We stopped. The girl stopped. I watched Barbara approach her again, and they sat down together in the tall grass. Christie walked slowly in our direction.

"What happened?" I asked her when she reached us.

"I'm not sure," she said. "Barbara found her lying next to a log at the back of the field, like she was hiding from someone. It's really sad. I've never seen anyone so scared."

The woman was sitting in the grass, her back to us. But I could see Barbara nodding, sometimes smiling, with every gesture, comforting. She reached out and put her arms around the woman and just held her for a few minutes, and I was reminded of once having heard that all we really want is for someone to put their arms around us and tell us that everything is going to be okay.

They stood up and faced the ambulance. Barbara nodded to me and I opened the door and stepped down into the grass. Christie and I walked forward to meet them, then helped the girl aboard. She refused to let go of Barbara.

"He's gonna be so mad," she said softly. She began to cry.

Barbara leaned toward the woman, establishing eye contact. "We talked about that, didn't we, Louise?" she said. "And we know that we've got to take care of you."

"Okay," she consented. "All right."

We drove back by the house, and Joe gave the thumbs-up to the deputy and we marked en route to Mary Washington Hospital.

The woman's blood pressure was very high, and she remained agitated throughout the trip to the hospital. She turned loose of Barbara reluctantly when we moved her to the stretcher in the emergency room.

I gave the ER nurse our report and walked out to the loading dock. Joe and Christie were getting a soda from the drink machine. Barbara was already on the ambulance.

"Hey — " I stuck my head inside the back of the ambulance — "that was a great job you did."

"Thank you," she said.

I saw that she was crying.

"Barbara," I said, climbing aboard. I sat next to her on the bench and put my arms around her.

"You're going to tell me everything's going to be all right, aren't you?" she said, smiling.

"No, I'm not," I said, returning her smile.

"Everybody ready?" Christie called to us from the front.

"Yeah, we're ready," I said, and Joe pulled away from the hospital.

"It just hurts so much," Barbara continued, "and it's so unfair."

I pulled away from her and reached in the cabinet for tissues and handed them to her.

"Thanks."

"Barbara, it is unfair and we see an awful lot of the unfairness. And it always hurts."

"What do you do?" she asked me.

"Well, first you have to decide if it's just too much pain, too much to deal with."

"Pat, I want to do this," she insisted. "I don't have any doubts about that. I just wondered what I, what anybody can do to make it hurt less."

"Do you know that your being with Louise helped to make it a little less unfair for her?"

"Do you think so?" she asked.

"Barbara, I know so. Why do you think she responded to you the way she did? She could tell how much you care. You may have been the only person to care about her for a long time. Don't you think that makes life a little better for her, that you were there?"

"Maybe so," she admitted.

"People tell us they are lucky because we are there to help them. I think we're the lucky ones, Barbara, because we're able to be there for a person at the time of their greatest need, to be able to help make things better, to help balance the unfairness.

"Try to think of it like that," I told her. "Try to remember."

Three

In 1909, on a bright, warm afternoon in southwestern Virginia, young Julian Wise strolled leisurely along the banks of the Roanoke River. He walked through flowering chicory and Queen Anne's lace down to the water's edge, slipped off his shoes, and sank his toes into the sandy river bottom.

A canoe drifted by, and the nine-year-old waved to the two men paddling it. They smiled and returned his wave, and he followed them with his gaze until they rounded a curve in the river. Then he dropped his shoes and waded in the shallows along the riverbank.

He heard the shouts before he reached the bend in the river, and hurried ahead to see what was happening.

The canoe had hit rapids and overturned in deep water. Far from the bank, the two men to whom Julian had waved only minutes before flailed their arms and shouted for help.

Others had heard the men and had come to the riverbank but they, like Julian, could do little more than watch. They had no rope, no boat, no strong swimmers. Some yelled advice. Others threw branches toward the men. But the branches fell far short.

The experience that day on the river stayed with Julian. He never forgot the sound of the men's desperate cries, the sight of them disappearing in the rough water, and the sudden stillness afterward. He never forgot his helplessness.

Several years later, he studied first aid with the Red Cross and Boy Scouts. Those sights and sounds and feelings still lingered in his mind, and he began to wonder how such a tragedy could have been prevented. He knew that first-aid training alone would not have been enough for him to have helped the men who died that day.

22

As Julian Wise grew into manhood, the question that had remained in his mind engendered an idea: What was needed was a squad of men trained in rescue techniques.

The idea expanded into a dream. And nineteen years after that tragic day on the Roanoke River, the dream became reality.

On May 28, 1928, Julian Wise and nine of his fellow workers at the Norfolk and Western Railway started the first volunteer rescue squad, the Roanoke life Saving and First Aid Crew.

At first, not too many people paid attention to the little band. Some were barely adults. All they had were bathing suits, a rowboat, and Wise's 1928 Dodge roadster. They answered only six calls that first year.

In 1986, Ed Wolfenden, one of the five surviving members of the original squad, told Brian O'Neill, reporter for the *Roanoke Times and World-News*, "Wise learned to mix shrewdness with his altruism. On a summer day in 1929, he got City Council's attention. He pulled off what would now be called a publicity stunt.

"Without telling other members of the squad," Wolfenden recalled, "Wise dumped an old suit full of rocks into Tinker Bell pool near Hollins. Then he called squad members at Norfolk and Western. They rushed to the scene. Council members were waiting.

"The squad dived to the simulated rescue. One fellow said, 'I found something down there but I couldn't move it.' The rock-filled dummy must have weighed 250 pounds," Wolfenden continued. "We found the durn thing right off the bat. Good gosh almighty, he didn't make it very realistic." It was realistic enough to get the council's attention.

Wise knew what he was doing. The city agreed to provide equipment and arranged for distress calls to go through the police and fire department switchboards. As the young men quickly proved themselves, public support began to grow. Oakey's Funeral Home donated a Cadillac ambulance and a round-the-clock driver. Squad membership expanded.

Wise's idea would catch on around the state, nation, and world as other communities saw the need for some organization specializing in providing emergency care. He actively promoted the volunteer rescue squad concept and estimated that he helped organize at least forty squads, earning him national recognition, including a citation in February 1973 from President Richard Nixon.

Nixon wrote of Wise: "The volunteer spirit has been one of the great strengths of American heritage, and your distinguished achievements demonstrate how much our nation has benefited from that tradition."

In July 1985, Julian Stanley Wise, who once said he wanted to be remembered for "giving people the advantage of knowing there's a rescue squad in their community," died at Lewis Gale Hospital in Salem, my home town. He was eighty-five years old.

In September of that year, the Virginia Association of Volunteer Rescue Squads celebrated its fiftieth anniversary at its annual convention in Roanoke. Tribute after tribute was paid to Wise, the founder and first president of the association.

A *Roanoke Times and World-News* editorial recalled Wise's unique contribution:

Neighbor helping neighbor is a practice that predates Western civilization. But helping in an emergency can require training and equipment that most people don't have. It was Wise's idea to incorporate the neighborly spirit, train those people willing to assist others, and keep their help accessible.

The volunteer can take a special pride in what he or she freely provides for other citizens. For those who come to need it, there can be no more valuable service. Julian Wise, whose efforts saved so many lives, finally gave his up this week. His work is his memorial.

In the years that followed that fateful day in May of 1928, the number of volunteer rescue squads continued to increase. The reality of Julian Wise's dream reached across America to cities and towns and outlying rural areas.

The service these squads provided prior to 1966 was invaluable, but limited. In many areas, it consisted solely of transportation to a medical facility. As a clearer understanding of what actually causes the body to die evolved, there also came the realization that if medical care were immediately available, some deaths previously considered inevitable would instead be preventable. The general agreement was that more prehospital care was needed.

A significant document that resulted in dramatic improvements in emergency medical services, *Accidental Death and Disability: The Neglected Disease of Modern Society*, was published in 1966 by the Division of Medical Services, National Academy of Science Research Council. This report stressed the difference that competent early emergency care could make in survival rates among the critically ill and injured.

A 1965 report from the President's Commission on Highway Safety had proposed emergency medical care and transportation of the sick and injured as one of its community action programs. This recommendation resulted in the inclusion of Standard 11, Emergency Medical Services, in the Highway Safety Act of 1966.

With passage of the Highway Safety Act, a closer look was taken at ambulance services, the majority of which still offered little more than transportation. Fewer than half of the estimated 200,000 ambulance and rescue personnel received training comparable to an advanced Red Cross level. Many had no training at all.

Only 465 of the 25,000 ambulances had the minimum equipment recommended by the American College of Surgeons. Only six states offered a standard training course for ambulance and rescue personnel, and none was equivalent to what is now considered "basic" training, the Emergency Medical Technician course.

The list of achievements in the first ten years following the Highway Safety Act was staggering. It included the establishment of training curriculum guidelines for EMTs, initiation of the EMT-Paramedic training course, emergency-vehicle design and equipment standards, state-coordinated training programs, improved communications and telemetry capabilities, a standard course on extrication from vehicle accidents, development of model emergency services systems, and official agencies in all state governments with delegated responsibility to administer and coordinate the emergency medical services program.

In April 1976, *The Journal of Trauma* published an article by Charles A. Rockwood, M.D., and associates, entitled "History of Emergency Medical Services in the United States." Its conclusion read: "The greatest threat to the average citizen in his own community today is not a fire in the home or a criminal in the street. The greatest threat is the inability to obtain adequate medical care at the time of need . . . when knowledge, skill, and minutes can save lives."

The Emergency Medical Services system is working to alleviate that threat. Recent gains made with the implementation of the Highway Safety Act and burgeoning medical technology have increased the effectiveness of emergency prehospital care.

Most patients who suffer fatal heart attacks die as the result of cardiac arrhythmias, disturbances in the rhythm of the heartbeat. These arrythmias can now be treated by prehospital personnel. Lives that once would have been lost on bedroom floors or in the backs of ambulances are now being saved by the administration of drugs and the use of a defibrillator.

Today, the survival rate of trauma patients is higher because of quick assessment and treatment, rapid fluid infusion and MAST trousers, and expedient transportation, often by medical-helicopter flight, to the nearest trauma center.

The growth of the Lake of the Woods Volunteer Rescue Squad paralleled the growth of other squads across the nation. In 1971, our ambulances carried Band-Aids and wooden splints. The equipment available now includes endotracheal tubes for advanced airway management and administration of life saving drugs, pulse oximeters to measure the patient's oxygen saturation level, and intraosseous infusion needles to enable rescue personnel to start IVs into the bone marrow of children.

In 1928, Julian Wise started the first volunteer rescue squad with ten men and a rowboat. Today, close to a half a million EMTs continue the service they began, incorporating the neighborly spirit, the training, and the accessibility of pre-hospital emergency care.

And, "for those who come to need it, there can be no more valuable service."

Four

My neighbor died last week. He was eighty-one years old.

I met him five years ago when he suffered his first heart attack. "Thank you for coming," he said to me when I took his hand in mine.

He was lying on the living room sofa — very still, but with a warmth that overwhelmed me, especially in the face of what he must have known was quite serious.

I rested my fingers on his radial pulse and could feel the irregularity. I could also feel the clamminess of his skin.

"Bob, on a scale of one to ten, what is the pain like?"

"A ten," he told me without hesitation.

"It started about an hour ago," Martha, his wife, said. "He was reading. He has angina, you know. He took a nitroglycerine. But it didn't do any good."

Joe wrote the information on the call sheet. He'd taken the man's blood pressure, 140 over 70. His pulse was 84, weak and irregular. His breaths were shallow. Paul put the non-rebreather oxygen mask on him. "This will help," he told Bob.

We hooked him up to the cardiac monitor and saw premature ventricular contractions, averaging twelve a minute, with some bigeminy. Joe set up an IV.

It was late at night, and the only light in the room was a soft reading lamp. Joe held a penlight so I could see to start the line. We called Mary Washington Hospital and requested orders for lidocaine, then gave a 75 mg bolus followed by a two-to-one drip. His blood pressure remained stable and we asked for morphine, since the nitroglycerine had done nothing for the pain. After 3 mg, the pain began to subside. By that time, the lidocaine had practically eliminated the PVCs.

Afterwards, he called us his angels.

He and his wife were people who brightened our days: good, loving people, the kind we need more of, not less. I saw Martha the day before Bob died. "He's out playing golf," she told me, smiling. "He feels great."

I heard the tones and the call, "Unresponsive male." I was pulling out of my driveway when the tones went off again for the same address; but, this time, the dispatcher announced, "CPR in progress."

"No," I whispered, a plea, a prayer.

When I reached the house, I gave Martha a quick embrace before I went to Bob. Art was already there. He had started CPR. Joe was ventilating with the bag mask. I placed the electrodes on Bob's chest. "V-fib, very fine." Mara reached for the paddles, then defibrillated twice. Asystole. I saw Martha watching us and asked Pia to go to her.

"Let's get him to the ambulance," I said to one of the others. Scott and Ricky helped move him quickly to the backboard, and within thirty seconds we were out the door and on the unit. Art stayed with Martha. Kirk continued the CPR. I started the IV and Bobby inserted an ET tube. Mara contacted Mary Washington Hospital. "Follow the protocol. We'll meet you at the loading dock," they told us.

We gave him all our epinephrine. And almost all our atropine.

On the monitor we saw the roller-coaster waves of Kirk's compressions. When I said, "Stop CPR" and Kirk lifted his hands off Bob's chest, the monitor showed only flatline.

Dr. Pennick met us on the loading dock. He checked the patency of the airway, the IV, and looked at the EKG summary. "Okay," he said — "I'm calling it."

I knew that if Bob could have been saved, we would have done it. I knew that.

Art brought Martha to the hospital and before we left, each of us went in to be with her for a few minutes. Mara and I knelt beside her and listened while she talked.

"He wouldn't have wanted to linger," she said to us. "He played eighteen holes of golf yesterday. And he won," she said, pausing briefly. "We were so lucky." She looked at me then and smiled, tears cresting in her eyes. "We had five extra years together. Lots of people don't have that, you know."

"I know," I told her.

A seasoned paramedic once said to me. "In EMS, there are two rules you have to remember. Rule number one is, people die. Rule number two is, you can't change rule number one."

It sounds so simple.

He was my mother's older brother, the joy of my grandmother's life, my grandfather's fair-haired boy, my Uncle Roy. He was a professor of history and he wrote a book about the law and he painted portraits in oil and he once ran for Congress in Virginia's Sixth District.

His last teaching job was at Western Virginia Community College, where students and faculty members began to lovingly call him "the absentminded professor." He joked about it himself as he occasionally forgot staff meetings, student appointments, and where he'd put exam papers. But as he remembered less and less, it was no longer funny. Still, it would be several years before we would learn that he was a victim of Alzheimer's disease.

He was not without his faults, but he was the only real Don Quixote I ever knew, and I watched him chase dreams and dragons and windmills.

His gifts to me were his laughter, the simplicity of his life, the strength of his spirit, and his passion for living.

It was Uncle Roy who introduced me to the Democratic Party.

My earliest election memory is going with my parents to their voting precinct in Salem and waiting for them while they cast their votes. My father wore his "I Like Ike" button.

I was a junior in high school when John Kennedy ran for President. My class was bused from Andrew Lewis High School to Woodrum Airport in Roanoke so we could see him. It was a clear and sunny day, and I was glad to be missing algebra class. Kennedy spoke for fifteen minutes, but I remembered little of what he said.

I was sitting at my desk on the campus of Bridgewater College studying for a French exam when he was assassinated. My room was on the second floor of Blue Ridge dorm. Someone from across the hall ran to my door and shouted, "The President's been shot."

The loss I felt was immense. And personal.

Then, in the spring of 1964, Uncle Roy told my parents he'd like to take me to Atlantic City for the Democratic National Convention. He was a national committeeman and could arrange for his daughter, my cousin Sandra, and me to sit on the convention floor with the delegates.

My parents of course said yes. "It's a wonderful opportunity," they told me. A week at the beach in Atlantic City certainly would be that, Sandra and I agreed. Uncle Roy was on the Platform Committee, so we arrived several days before the convention actually began. We were asked to be Young Citizens for Johnson, which meant we got to wear red, white, and blue LBJ smocks around town. We were nineteen years old and feeling important.

On the opening night, we took our places near the Virginia delegation. We saw Walter Cronkite and Howard K. Smith in their booths high above the stage. During the week Peter, Paul, and Mary serenaded us, and we listened to speeches from Birch Bayh and Paul Newman and Hubert Humphrey. It was Humphrey who first got my attention, who made Sandra and me realize that Convention Hall was perhaps a more important place to be than the boardwalk. There, we met the Mississippi Freedom Delegation, and outside, on the steps, I shook hands with Dr. Martin Luther King.

On Wednesday night, Bobby Kennedy stepped up to the podium to speak, and the mere sight of him brought everyone on the convention floor to their feet. The crowd cheered for twenty minutes. We cheered for Bobby and for Jack; we cheered for America and the world. And for ourselves. That night, I think we salvaged a little of what we'd all lost in Dallas on that cold November day.

Uncle Roy introduced me to politics. He was the first person who ever really discussed issues with me. He gave me books to read; he picked my brain, and let me pick his. He helped me open my eyes wider, and then he showed me places to look.

My parents taught me about commitment and altruism, about fairness and decency and God. They taught me to always leave a place better than I find it, to never judge, and to always stand up for what I think is right.

Uncle Roy was passionate about life. That was his legacy to me.

Over four million Americans suffer from title cruel disease called Alzheimer's, a progressive, degenerative disease that results in impaired memory, thinking, and behavior; and, finally, death. After heart disease, cancer, and stroke, it is the fourth leading cause of death in adults in the United States, claiming more than 100,000 lives annually.

All of them, when their minds were whole and unencumbered, added joy and life to those who loved them, as Uncle Roy did for me.

Her name was Pearl. His was Edward. They lived in our community, a short three blocks apart. They never met; but if they had, neither would have remembered the other. Pearl was fifty-eight when she died and Edward was sixty-five, but I believe they died long before their hearts gave out.

Pearl's daughter took care of her. Most of our calls for Pearl were for "general weakness." She was basically strong and healthy, as is the case with many Alzheimer's patients. It is a slow deterioration of the mind, and then of the body. In the final stages, patients with Alzheimer's wear diapers and their frail bodies curl into the fetal position.

Calls for Edward were primarily search parties. While his daughter was at work and he was under the care of a housekeeper, he would sometimes just walk away. Twice, we found him deep in the woods. Once, he was sitting on a neighbor's front porch: he thought he was home.

I got to know Edward's daughter, and Pearl's. Pearl's daughter cared not just for Pearl, but for her own husband, who had cancer. Edward's daughter was a single parent with two children. Both houses had night lights in every room, gates to block stairways, and double locks on all outside doors.

Pearl and Edward were not our only Alzheimer's patients. Some people with Alzheimer's disease are involved in automobile accidents, as passengers and drivers. Others, like Edward, become disoriented and lose their way, and we have to find them. Some are violent.

Others have other medical problems. All are so very, very sad. Not only are they ill; they are trapped in their illness and held prisoners by their minds.

"We don't know for sure," the doctors at the Veterans Administration Hospital in Salem had told my mother, Uncle Roy's wife, Elsa, and Marsha, Uncle Roy's other daughter. "There is no single test we can do to identify Alzheimer's."

Elsa and Uncle Roy had met in the Canal Zone when he was serving as the director of the Florida State University Extension there. They married in 1966 and moved to Roanoke, where he taught history and political science. Following his departure from his teaching post at Virginia Western Community College, they returned to Panama to live. At first, we communicated fairly often. Then his letters came less and less frequently.

In the summer of 1986, my parents called me and told me Uncle Roy and Elsa were coming to Salem. And they told me why.

They admitted him to the Veterans Hospital for tests. They gave him a thorough physical examination including neurological and mental-status assessments. They did blood studies, urinalysis, electrocardiograms, electroencephalograms, chest X-rays, and a spinal tap to examine the cerebrovascular fluid.

A week later, the doctors reported that while confirmation of Alzheimer's requires an examination of brain tissue, usually performed at an autopsy, they were prepared to say that Uncle Roy did, indeed, suffer from Alzheimer's disease.

I drove to Salem the day he was released from the hospital, I hadn't seen him for six years, and he and Elsa were leaving that day to return to Panama. Somehow, we misunderstood the schedule, and almost missed them.

Our only hope was that Mickey Overstreet, who lived next to my parents and worked for Piedmont Airlines, could delay the departure. He radioed the pilot and then accompanied us out to the runway. When the stewardess told us they couldn't hold the plane, Mickey told her, "It's not leaving until they have a chance to go aboard for a few minutes,"

Mama and I walked down the narrow aisle of the plane. I spotted them and took her hand. "There they are," I said.

"Don't be long," Mickey reminded us.

Uncle Roy had the aisle seat, Elsa the window. I knelt beside him and put my arms around him. "I've missed you," I said, my face nestled against his sweater. He was so thin. I leaned back to look closely at his face.

He patted my arm. "It was nice of you to come," he said, slowly, almost methodically.

He didn't even know me.

I looked up at my mother, then at Elsa. Elsa glanced away.

"Roy," my mother said, her voice breaking, "you remember Patricia."

"Patricia?" he said, looking at her, not me. "Yes, Patricia."

"Edna, we have to go," Mickey said to my mother.

"Uncle Roy," I said, softly. He looked at me, then. But it was a stare, really, just an empty, vacant stare.

I never saw him again.

On June 19, 1989, six days before his seventy-third birthday, his heart finally, mercifully, gave out. He died with Elsa beside him in the home they shared in Boquete, Chiriquí, in the Republic of Panama.

Just across the bridge over the Rapidan River that separates Orange and Culpeper Counties, on a little triangle of land between Route 3 and Route 610, sits a country store called Germanna Gas 'n Stuff. Carl and Laurie Johnson own it. They sell all the staples that you'd find in a modern convenience store, plus fresh meat on Tuesdays. And you can't find a better bacon, lettuce, and tomato sandwich anywhere.

They bought the store in 1987 and fixed it up themselves. The day they called the rescue squad, Carl had been putting up a new exterior wall, and it had fallen on him.

The lunch crowd had the wall off him when we arrived. He was lying very still and complaining of pain in his ankle and his right little finger. After our assessment, which revealed a fractured ankle and finger and some small lacerations on the top of his head, Norm and Jack put the cervical collar on him. Pia and I used a pillow splint for his ankle, and we bandaged his head. Then we logrolled him onto the backboard.

Everything had gone pretty smoothly up until that point. He was in good spirits, and the lunch crowd assured him the wall was in good shape. I got on the ambulance to help guide the gurney in. Norm and Pia and Jack were at the foot of the gurney when Pia somehow got her finger caught.

She yelled, startling all of us, including Carl.

We had to take the gurney back off the ambulance and work Pia's finger out from between the narrow bars. It was already turning blue.

"Pia," I told her, "you get on and I'll help them with the gurney. Then I'll get you some ice."

"Is everything okay?" Carl asked. His head was taped to the backboard and it was hard for him to see anywhere but straight above him.

"Oh, yeah," Norm assured him. "Everything's fine."

Again we started to ease him onto the ambulance.

And a bug flew into my eye.

"Oh!" I exclaimed.

"What?" Norm responded.

"Nothing," I answered him, one eye tightly shut.

The gurney latched in. "Is everything all right?" Carl asked.

"Well, Carl," Norm said, "if this keeps up you may have to get up and let one of us lie down."

Carl smiled nervously, but I don't think he thought it was very funny.

Jack drove to Culpeper Memorial Hospital and Norm took care of Carl. I wrapped an ice pack around Pia's finger and then, with her good hand, she got the bug out of my eye.

Five

O N July 22, 1985, five hours after Julian Wise died, a call came into the Roanoke Life Saving and First Aid Crew. "Roanoke River. Possible drowning." The responding crew found a thirteen-year-old boy who was unconscious and had aspirated water into his lungs.

And they saved him.

Things had come full circle.

In 1909, Julian Wise had witnessed a drowning in the Roanoke River. The young boy survived on that July day seventy-six years later because Julian Wise had had a vision and had turned that vision into a reality.

In August 1985, a month after Julian died, Roanoke's Mayor Noel Taylor recommended in his State of the City address that a museum and national headquarters for volunteer rescue squads be established in Roanoke. In 1988, the Julian Stanley Wise Foundation was formed to design and raise money for the volunteer rescue exhibition. The site they chose far the museum was a three thousand-square-foot wing of the Roanoke Valley History Museum, located on the third level of the Center in the Square Cultural Complex.

The Foundation then hired Conover Hunt as a consultant. As executive director of the Dallas Historical Society Association, Conover had been the creative force in the Kennedy Museum (The Sixth Floor) in the Book Depository in Dallas, Texas. She brought experience and creative enthusiasm to the "To The Rescue" project, and was the first to recognize its national possibilities.

It took almost three years from inception to completion. On June 8, 1991, "To The Rescue" opened to great fanfare. Fifty ambulances from around the Commonwealth of Virginia and beyond paraded from the old Roanoke Life Saving and First Aid Crew building to Center in the Square.

Ceremonies included a message of congratulations from President Bush, delivered by Theresa Miller of the White House Office of National Service, and one from the National Highway Safety Administration. James McGuire, president of the Virginia Association of Volunteer Rescue Squads, welcomed the crowd to the grand opening. The guest of honor was Julian's widow, Ruth Light Wise. At promptly two o'clock, Dan Hall, Fire Chief of the Salem Fire Department, rang the bell marking the official opening.

"This is the nation's first permanent museum display devoted to the history of emergency medical and rescue services," the executive director of the Wise Foundation, David Murray, exclaimed. His exuberance was reminiscent of Conover's. "Not everyone has vision, you know," he said to me.

"I know," I agreed. We were standing together in the museum, and we had to speak loudly to each other to be heard above the crowd.

"Julian had vision," he said.

We paused at the first exhibit, a theatrical staging — a Mazda GLC crashed into a wall. The car rested on its roof, one tire still spinning, the driver partially ejected. It was a dramatic introduction to the world of emergency medicine. Next to it was a telephone, over which, when we dialed 911, we could hear a woman reporting to the dispatcher the accident we had just witnessed.

Dave and I moved together through the museum, greeting friends, pausing to view the videos depicting the spirit of volunteerism, and showing dramatic footage of actual rescues — the most memorable one being the rescue of baby Jessica. They were stirring images, and all who watched them were visibly moved. I was surrounded by men and women from volunteer rescue squads, and as we watched the screens we shared the same emotions. We were not there when Jessica was pulled from the well, but each of us had been at another place, another time, the site of another tragedy involving a baby Jessica. Tears stung our eyes as we remembered the triumphant moments, the moments of defeat.

"This museum is for all of you," Conover said to me. She was vibrant. She had watched this project from its beginning. "I really understand now what it is you people do," she said, smiling, and I believed her. She took my hand and led me toward the next exhibit. "Look at the crash truck." We climbed inside. "Put your seat belt on," she told me. As soon as we did, a video began. Displayed across the front windshield, the video portrayed an actual drive to a rescue scene. "I have to take my Dramamine before I watch this one," she laughed.

The museum includes artifacts from twenty-six states and three foreign countries. There is a plaque dedicated to the volunteers who have lost their lives. "We never had a place to honor the volunteers lost in the line of duty," Mac McGuire commented. "We give more than just our time," he added solemnly. "And these people gave everything."

In 1934, six years after Julian Wise started the first volunteer squad, he was asked why it had been so important to him. He replied, "I resolved that I was going to become a lifesaver and that never again would I watch a man die when he could have been saved if only those around him knew how."

I have been an EMT instructor since 1988. And I begin each new class with that quotation. I tell them that I am proud of the commitment they have made and that for the rest of their lives, those around them will be safer, will have a better chance of beating the odds, because they will have the knowledge and the skills to save them.

In each new class, we talk briefly about why we are there. "I once was afraid of blood," I tell them. "And look at me now," I smile. "Training displaces fear. So when there is an emergency, we have something to draw on other than being afraid or repulsed. We are more prepared for the unexpected."

I became a cardiac technician in 1984, and the next year I decided it would be a good idea to sit in on an EMT class to refresh my basic skills. I walked into the classroom that first night and took a chair near the back. The instructor sat at a table in front of the room, reading. He didn't look up from his book until five minutes after the class was to begin.

He stood up then and f aced the twenty-three people. "Half of you people won't finish this class," he said, "because you don't have what it takes."

I went back the next week, just to see. He was right. Half of them didn't have what it took. I counted eleven people.

I think of that EMT class each time I begin with a new group of people. I hear their muffled voices and their footsteps on the stairs as they climb to the second-floor classroom. I see the skepticism, the self-doubts on many faces that first night. And I watch them closely as we move through the chapters of the book — head and chest injuries, shock, childbirth, pediatrics, and heart attacks.

Together, we find humor in small things, because laughter is good for us all, and we must find humor where we can. And we say "good job" to each other when the bandage is snug and when the splint has immobilized the arm.

I watch their faces on the night I teach them how to take a patient's blood pressure. A cuff is a cuff, I tell them. You don't have to call it a sphygmomanometer. Stethoscope tips in the ears correctly, locate the brachial pulse, make sure the cuff is the right size . . . pump . . . release. . . . Then there's excitement on each face. "Yes, I heard it!" they exclaim.

"Good job! "I tell them all.

In 1989, my first class of EMTs graduated. They were my "Grubnelednerts." Lester Brim coined that one when we studied shock. The position in which to put a patient who is going into shock is with the feet raised, and is called the Trendelenburg position.

Lester waved his hand in the air. "Pat," he said excitedly, "do you know what 'Trendelenburg' spelled backwards is?" And before any of us had a chance to think or to answer, he announced, "Grubnelednert!"

On graduation night, they gave me a pin to wear, with the inscription, "Number One Grubnelednert." And I gave them a poem entitled "To My EMTS":

We've studied and practiced and studied some more,
And your friends say, "Gosh, you've become such a bore
With your talk of KEDS and something called MAST.
Will it ever be over — How long will it last?"
"Quite a long time," you just might have said
For all of this knowledge is now in your head.

Not just to be there tucked deeply away,
But instead, for a purpose, to be used night or day.

Now you know there are 27 bones in the hand.
And you don't think of marine life when you hear SHRIMP CAN.
Burns you know, first, second, and third degree —
And you know that the patella is really the knee.

Ecchymosis is just a big word for bruise
And to get a pedal pulse you must first remove the shoes.
Diabetic Coma is not at all like Insulin Shock.
Anterior hip dislocation — one foot in the boat and one on the dock.

Cover both eyes — the left and the right.
Don't forget to report all animal bites.
Don't induce vomiting if the culprit is lye,
And don't ever be ashamed to cry.

You can save someone's life with your knowledge and skill,
Give someone hope — give someone the will
To keep on through even the darkest time
When life seems to have lost its rhythm and rhyme,
With the warmth of your smile and the touch of your hand,
With your eyes that say, "I understand."

There are just no words to express the way
I feel about you — Purvis, John, Hunter and Jay,
Sally, Andi, and Debbie and Tommy and Mac.
It goes much deeper than a pat on the back.

For Sandy, Millie, and Linnea, the feeling's the same . . . As with
Norm, Paul, and Mike, Lester and Larry — you ALL
deserve fame.
We'll be together through joys and hurts.
We're bonded — We're the GRUBNELEDNERTS!

And so my EMTs, this is our last night here,
Where all of you, to me, have grown so dear.

Go now from this room where we've learned so much
About emergency care and the magic of touch.

More than medical skills I've tried to impart;
Remember, the brain cannot work without the heart.

I gave them gold stars when they scored high on their tests. I gave them valentines in February and tiny stockings with peppermint sticks at Christmas. I watched them grow and become the best they could be. And I would be with many of them in the years to come.

I was with Sally on her first rescue call and the night she gave birth to her son. Purvis joined the crew with Joe and Norm and me. Linnea served briefly, then moved to Ohio with her family. Andi, too, was with us a short time. Tommy became captain of the Richardsville Rescue Squad. Jay, Joe's son, ran calls until his own accident. Millie serves as a CPR instructor. Debbie became a cardiac technician and went to work in the emergency room in Alexandria Hospital.

Mac and Paul and Norm were not new EMTs. Each was recertifying. In June 1992, we surprised Mac with a celebration in honor of his twenty years of service on the squad. Paul will be next. He has served sixteen. And, Norm, my dear Norm: in spring 1991, we saved his life.

That was my first EMT class. They were the Grubnelednerts.

My very first students met in a classroom in rural Rockingham County, Virginia, over twenty years ago. It was a class of sixteen four and five-year-old Head Start students. Each day was an adventure for them as we worked and played together, and it was in that Shenandoah Valley school that I learned about the magic of touch and how vital it is to learning.

They were eager to count to a hundred, to know what stars are made of, to figure how far it is to California, and to learn why blue and yellow turn to green. We learned all about colors in the leaves and in rainbows and in fingerpaint. They were beginning to love learning. I was beginning to love them, their little upturned faces, their smiles of sunshine and their small hands, sticky with perspiration and peanut butter, reaching for mine.

For they also wanted to hold on to someone, to feel they were a part of something bigger, to hear a voice say, "That's so good," when their pictures were taped on the wall.

"You are very special," I would always tell them.

Adults aren't so different, when it comes to teaching them. Their minds, perhaps, are not quite as open or pliable. Ideas and thought processes have taken shape and jelled. But hearts are the same, I think. And everyone likes Christmas candy canes. And gold stars and valentines still bring smiles.

Six

Like me, Holly is an only child. Perhaps that is one reason why we blossom in this extended family.

"She was looking for a place where she could make a difference," Lester, her husband of five years, told me. His pride in her was apparent. "A place where she could be appreciated," he added.

Because of job pressures, Lester was unable to commit himself to the squad. But he added "Grubnelednert" to our EMT vocabulary, and he made us laugh when we needed it the most.

"I think she initially became interested in the squad because I was," he said. "Then she realized that 'hey, this is something I can do.'"

The odor of blood, acrid and heavy, met them at the doorway.

"It was overpowering," Holly told me later over the phone. "They think he'd probably been dead for several hours."

Bobby and Purvis and Holly were on duty when the call for "a possible suicide" came in. "Possible suicide" is too little information for me. I want to know more. I want to know, was a note found? Was a person found? Did a neighbor report the sound of gunshots? Is there a handful of pills missing, a rope swinging from an attic rafter, a car left running in a closed garage? Tell us more.

Don't let us walk unaware into a house reeking of blood.

"The deputy was already there," Holly said. "He walked in with us, through the living room, and down the hall. It was so eerie. There was no furniture in the house except for the sofa where the man was sitting and a small table in front of him with pictures of his wife and his son.

"I stood behind him," Holly continued, "while Bobby and Purvis and the deputy checked him. He just looked asleep," she said. "From

42

where I stood, I couldn't see his chest, so it just looked like he'd fallen asleep."

"I didn't want to look," she told me.

"I don't blame you, Holly," I said. "I wouldn't have wanted to look, either."

The suicide note was on the table next to the pictures. Short and to the point. "I don't want to live alone."

He was only twenty-eight years old.

"I don't want to live alone . . ."

Emptiness. Empty house. Empty beer cans. Empty fifth of vodka. Empty bottle of Dilantin. Empty chambers in the double-barrel shot gun.

His parents, who lived nearby, had begun to worry when there was no answer to their phone calls. They were sitting in their pickup truck in front of their son's house when the crew arrived.

"The father found him. Won't let the mother in," the deputy said to Holly as they walked down the empty hallway. "Can't blame him for that," he said, slowly shaking his head.

He was their only child.

"I'll be here if you need anything," I told her.

"I know," she said. "A lot of it is just sorting things through."

We said good-bye.

It was weeks later on a Sunday afternoon. We were in the rescue bay together updating the bulletin board.

"Is everything okay, Holly?" She'd been unusually quiet.

"I think so," she said.

"Not good enough," I smiled at her. "Put those thumb tacks down," I said, "and let's have a seat."

We climbed on the ambulance. I sat in the jump seat. Holly sat on the bench and propped her feet up on the gurney. She leaned her head back and I could see her eyes were moist with tears.

"At first," she said softly, "I didn't even know what I was feeling. I anticipated sadness or depression but it didn't happen. It was my worst call and I couldn't get through it because I couldn't figure out what I was dealing with.

"It was awful," she continued. "The father was trying so hard to hold his emotion in. The mother was guilt-ridden and kept crying. 'If only we'd come sooner.' Then he would say to her over and over, 'It's not our fault. It's not our fault.'"

"It must have been awful, Holly."

She nodded. "When I think of those parents, my heart breaks."

She pushed strands of her strawberry-colored hair away from her face. "It was anger," she said softly.

So softly I didn't understand what she'd said.

"What?" I asked.

"Anger," she repeated. "I finally realized it was anger I was feeling. Anger at him for the destruction he'd caused, the terrible damage he'd done, the guilt and anguish of his parents. And who knows what effect this will have on his wife and on his son?"

We talked for more than an hour that day in the back of the ambulance about anger and fear and sadness and loss, and hope. I told her that the parents were lucky to have her there, to have her comfort and her love.

Holly is okay now.

But I sometimes worry. I have encouraged these people to join the rescue squad and I have taught them to be EMTs. I have measured them for new uniforms and assigned them to duty crews.

I try to keep them safe.

Make sure the scene is safe, I tell them. Certain calls demand law enforcement — shootings, stabbings, suicides, overdoses. If we're uncertain about the scene being secure, we ask for a deputy. We've never been hurt badly on a call. There've been little things — Pia smashed her finger; I fell on the floor when the ambulance stopped suddenly; half of us have hurt our backs at one time or another; we get small cuts sometimes from protruding metal and shards of glass at auto accidents.

I don't worry so much about physical injury. Most of the time, we're careful. It's long-term emotional injury I sometimes fear.

"It doesn't go away that easily," Leroy told me. We talk often. For me, he's something of a touchstone. "You remember the walkway that collapsed in the hotel in Kansas City?"

"Oh yes," I told him.

"Well, the medical personnel who worked that were involved in several debriefings, and most of them seemed okay. Years passed, and then recently, some of the people who were there agreed to be a part of a video on the importance of debriefing. They thought it was all behind them. Then they started talking about it, and the more they talked, the more they remembered, and after a while, for some of them it seemed like the accident was just yesterday."

"Is there any way to prevent that?" I asked him.

"Not really," he admitted. "I think it's important to just keep talking. Have a support group, someone you're close to. And realize, even though you can force things out of your mind, it's never going to completely go away. Certain things will always trigger it."

And I remembered Kirk's words: "Whenever I clean the chimney in my house, I remember. The smell . . . the smell brings it back."

It was a cold Sunday morning in November. I got up at 5:45, brushed my teeth, and went to the bathroom. I pulled my nightshirt off over my head and put on my bra and a turtleneck shirt; then, trying not to open my eyes too wide, I sat on the side of my bed and put on my socks. My uniform, unzipped and ready for me to slip into, was hanging on the bathroom shower rod. My tennis shoes were on the floor beneath my uniform, tongues folded back for quick entry.

It was 5:54. I would go on duty in six minutes, and I was ready. Back when I was a very new EMT, I would get up at 5:00 and take a shower, put on my uniform, and wait. By three in the afternoon, I'd be dozing off. I ran with Ed Law then — he'd show up on early morning calls with his pajamas hanging out the bottom of his uniform. It didn't take me long to see the advantages of his way of thinking.

I reset my alarm for 7:30 and got back into bed.

At 6:26 the tones went off: "A 1050, overturned vehicle."

So much for a quiet Sunday morning.

The call was a mile west on Route 3. Norm had the ambulance out when I arrived. Joe pulled in just behind me. We marked en route to the scene with a fire engine behind us.

"Any further information?" I asked the dispatcher.

"Overturned trailer," she said. "Broke away from the vehicle towing it. No hazardous materials. That's all we've got."

Moments later, we arrived on the scene.

At our 1990 annual banquet, this was the call to which we paid honor. Here are the highlights of the poem I wrote dedicated to our "Super Seven" firemen:

The Saga Of The Super Seven

It was six thirty in the morning and most were asleep.
But not Fire and Rescue . . . we had promises to keep.
For fate had fallen cruelty on some traveling passers-by,
And as we neared the accident scene we heard the muffled cry.
Our vehicle bore proudly the star of blue and white,
Our beacon glowed for all to see — the red rotating light.
Joe and Norm and I moved quickly — we knew just what to do,
As we stumbled through the briers, trying to reach Patients One and Two.
Their vehicle was overturned. Upon its top it lay.
"I don't know." "Doesn't look too good," we heard bystanders say.
We peered inside the wreckage, saw legs and hair and shoes,
For there, there trapped inside, were Patients One and Two.
We were armed with oxygen, stethoscope, and BP cuff,
A KED, HARE Splint, MAST; and if that weren't enough . . .
. . . we'd start a line with Ringers if the BP began to fall.
Trained and skilled EMTs, we give our patients our all.
We glanced at each other and then looked back at One and Two,
Then sadly shook our heads and sighed . . . We'd met our Waterloo!
We can handle strokes and heart attacks. We can handle trauma, too.
But we'd never seen anything like the likes of Patients One and Two.
We knew then we'd have to call a doctor who knew about such things,
And in the hamlet of Stephensburg, that doctor's phone would ring.

He hurried to the accident scene with medical bag in hand.

"For Patients One and Two," he said, "I'll do everything I can."

But it wasn't enough. More had to be done for Patients One and Two.

It was a moment for heroes; but where would we find such courage tried and true?

And then the Super Seven stepped forward in their yellow turnout gear,

And what they did was incredible — the extrication of the year.

Their sounding trumpet was a generator that burst forth with a blast;

For Patients One and Two, the Super Seven would work hard and they'd work fast.

Bill and Bobby cribbed. John and Kevin got the Halogen bar.

Dan and Chief Jack held the Jaws of Life as we watched them from afar.

Then I saw Captain Ferguson walk slowly away from Squad 29;

He walked straight and tall toward the wreckage. And how his eyes did shine.

He looked back once and smiled broadly, then nodded a time or two.

And we knew right then that all would be fine for Patients One and Two.

And the tool that he had there sparkled in the early morning sun,

As he set off through briers and brambles to finally get the job done.

It was the magical saw that cuts through steel that he carried on his hip;

The magical saw with the carbide blade and the polished diamond tip.

And he stood before the vehicle that still on its top lay,

And he powered the saw we call K-12 and proceeded to save the day.

The clangor and clamor of the saw exploded in the morning air;

And we held our breath knowing that we were almost there.

And as the K-12 was cutting through that vehicle on the ground,

Sparks burst forth from that diamond-tipped blade and there came a thundering sound.

And we all stood back in wonder while through the doors they galloped through,

When Captain Ferguson lit the spark under Patients One and Two.

Now, for you who've listened to this saga and are wondering what's all the to-do;

It's that Patient One was a brown quarter horse and the gray was Patient Two.

And the Super Seven were the heroes of the brown quarter horse and the gray,

And, all in all, it turned out to be a most remarkable day.

The duty crew was out on a call for a man who'd fallen on a patch of ice when the second call came in. This time it was "difficulty breathing." Bill was the only one there when I arrived at the building.

"I guess it's just you and me," I told him. "Let's go." I let the dispatcher know we were en route, undermanned, with a cardiac technician and a driver.

The call was in Culpeper County. Richardsville's Company Six was already on the scene. Gary met us in the driveway.

"Hey, Pat," he said, taking the cardiac monitor from me as I stepped off the ambulance. It was bitterly cold, and we hurried toward the house. "She's having a lot of trouble breathing and it's really hard getting a pulse. Tommy and Jan are with her."

The woman was in her bedroom in the back of the house. She smiled at me when I walked in the door, but it was a sad smile.

The room was like a furnace and she had on a heavy fur-lined coat. Jan was on the bed with the woman trying to help her sit up. I sat down beside her. Her breaths were shallow, labored.

"Are you having any pain or pressure in your chest?" I asked her. She shook her head.

"When did this start?"

"This morning," she said. I glanced at my watch: four-thirty. Why did she wait so long?

"You have your coat on. Were you going somewhere?" I asked her.
"To the doctor," she said. The smile was fixed. Her eyes were glassy, vacuous.

Jan held the oxygen mask up to her face. "Try to slow your breathing," she told her. "The oxygen will help."

"Does she live alone?" I asked Jan.

"No, we called her husband at work. He's going to meet us at the hospital. He said she wasn't feeling well this morning."

"What's her history?"

"Diabetes and congestive heart failure," Jan answered me.

Tommy and I struggled to get her coat off. She lay back against Jan while I loosened her blouse to place the electrodes on her chest. Perspiration was running down my face, and the perspiration on her was so heavy, the electrodes wouldn't stick. It was hard to tell if the diaphoresis was from the temperature in the house or from her medical condition.

"I can feel a weak radial pulse," Tommy said. "It's really irregular."

"Let's get her on the gurney," I said. "We just can't do anything in this heat." Gary and Bill lifted her on the gurney. Jan slipped the non-rebreather mask on her face.

I carried the lifepack out to the ambulance. I'd get everything set up there, and then when they got her on . . .

"Pat," Jan yelled from the back of the ambulance, "she's stopped breathing."

"Get her up here," I said.

They pushed the gurney onto the unit. She was still sitting. Her eyes remained open, glazed. "Put her down and get the board," I said. Tommy lowered the head of the gurney. I ventilated twice and then checked for a carotid.

"No pulse." Bill slipped the CPR board under her.

"Gary, start CPR. Jan, get the bag mask."

Her eyes closed. She was in asystole and stayed in asystole until they called the code fifteen minutes after we arrived at the hospital.

"It was awful," I told Joe later. He'd been on an earlier call, and had only heard snatches of our conversations with the dispatcher and the hospital. He was at the building when we got back. "Everything went wrong."

"Why don't you think of the things that went right?" he asked me.

I just shook my head. "Because nothing did." I was finishing the paper work. "I have to keep a copy for the report for Dr. Kravetz since, as Bill puts it, she died on our watch."

"Something must have gone right," he persisted.

I turned and faced him. "Well, if you're looking for something that went right, we didn't run out of gas. But we couldn't get anything done in the house because it was so hot. The patches wouldn't stay on. She was so wet I couldn't get a quick look I trusted. So," I sighed, "I just didn't have a handle on what was happening.

"I was the only one in the unit familiar with it. Tommy and Jan and Gary were great but they weren't used to our ambulance. Her veins were so bad I couldn't get an IV started.

"Then, we get to the hospital and her husband is there waiting for us. Of course, when he last saw her she was alive . . . and now, she's dead. Now, you see what I mean?"

"Yeah," he nodded. "I see what you mean." He put his arm on my shoulder and pulled me close to him. "It'll be all right," he said.

"Sure," I said, sounding halfhearted, but knowing he was right.

Because he always makes me believe it will be.

Seven

Looking back, Ithink both of us knew we weren't going to make it across the creek.

The man on horseback was ahead, leading us down a narrow logging trail to the place where his wife had been thrown from her horse. "Her neck's hurt bad," was all he'd said when he met us at the road.

His horse waded effortlessly across the creek. I looked at Joe. "You think we can make it?" I asked.

"Probably."

"I don't know," I said, watching the man on horseback round a bend in the trail. "How much further did he say she was?"

"A half a mile," Joe answered.

The front wheels dropped into the creek and Joe accelerated. They moved easily up the opposite side. He sighed. "Halfway there."

Then the back wheels dropped in. And stayed.

"Hmmm."

He looked at me. "Don't say it."

"How much further did he say she was?" I asked.

"About a half a mile."

I opened the door. "Okay," I said, "I'm going to take a collar and some four-by-fours and cling and the radio."

"Take them where?" he asked.

"I'm going to follow the man," I told him.

"You don't even know where he went."

"Well, I can't just sit here. I saw him go around that bend, right up there," I said, pointing toward the hill. "I'll just follow the trail."

"Okay," he agreed. "I guess I should see about getting this ambulance out of here."

I stuffed bandages and cling in my pockets, carried the collar in one hand and the radio in the other. "I'll let you know what's happening."

I tried to find a spot where the creek narrowed some but didn't see a spot in either direction. I stepped in the water, then onto the opposite side. "I'm off in search of my knight on horseback."

He laughed. "Just be careful."

"I will," I called over my shoulder. "Just get our ambulance out of the creek."

I continued up the hill. I waved to Joe when I reached the bend, then rounded it. "Portable 291 to Med 291," I said into the radio.

"Go ahead," Joe answered.

"Radio check," I said. "How do you copy?"

"Loud and clear."

Good. I could easily reach him. I rounded another bend and saw just ahead that the trail divided. When I reached the fork, I stopped. "Okay," I said softly to myself. "What now?"

Suddenly I heard a noise from deep in the woods, footsteps on leaves, branches breaking. I turned and looked toward the trees.

It's all downhill back to the ambulance, I thought to myself. I could yell into the radio and just start running now and get away from whatever's coming out of the woods . . .

It was the man on his horse!

"What are you doing in the woods?" I asked him. I was trying very hard to sound totally in control while my knees were about to buckle.

"I took the shortcut back," he said, looking up and down the trail. "Where is your ambulance?"

"Well," I said, "it's in the creek."

"My wife can barely move and your ambulance is in the creek?"

"He's getting it out and I'm going with you," I said. "I'm sorry, but right now that's the best we can do."

"I guess you're right." He nudged his horse with his heels and she turned back onto the trail. "Well, follow me."

"How much further?" I asked him.

"At least three quarters of a mile," he said.

"I thought we were almost there."

"Nope."

The trail was almost all uphill. My legs were beginning to feel heavy.

"Why don't you ride ahead," I suggested, "and check on your wife. I'd like to know how she's doing since we're still pretty far away."

He turned a little in his saddle and looked back at me. "What do you want me to do?" he asked.

"Just check on her. Make sure she's breathing okay. I don't like her being alone up here."

"She's not alone," he said. "The dogs are with her. But if you think I should go, maybe I should."

"I do," I told him. "And I'll be there as soon as I can. Oh — " I called to him " — are there any more forks in the road?"

"Nope, it's a straight shot," he answered.

Again, I was alone. I glanced at my watch. I'd been on this trail for twenty minutes. I looked behind me. No sign of the ambulance.

"Portable 291 to 291," I said into the radio.

No answer.

"Portable 291 to 291."

"This is 291," Joe said.

"Are you en route?" I asked.

"Negative," he responded. He sounded pretty deflated. "Not yet."

"I haven't reached the scene," I told him. "This road is really awful. When you come up the hill, bear right at the fork."

"Okay," was all he said.

"It's not going well, "I mumbled, shaking my head. "Not well at all."

Joe had found a small shovel in the tool box on the ambulance. He was trying to dig out a path with that while he waited for the crash truck to respond when a man named John Gentry pulled up behind him in his pickup truck.

"Gonna take a long time with that," he said, getting out of his truck. Gentry lived less than a mile away. We'd passed his house just before we turned onto the logging trail. He'd gotten curious and decided to see what was going on. "I got a backhoe at home. I could go get it."

Joe stood up and faced him.

"You may have just saved my life."

"Yeah," he nodded. "I imagine you'd be in some trouble if that thing floated downstream."

"To say the least," Joe admitted.

"Don't worry, buddy," John said, stepping into his truck. "We'll get it out."

I stopped for a minute just to catch my breath. The victim's husband rode back down the path toward me. "She's not doing too good," he said.

"What do you mean?"

"Well, she says she's having trouble moving her hands, they're numb. Her head really hurts and her neck. And I think her nose is broken." Again, he looked down the trail. "Where the hell is that ambulance?"

"Look," I said, "I can assure you that we'll take care of her and get her to the hospital."

He shook his head. "I don't see how, with no ambulance."

"Sir, believe me, we will. The ambulance is almost clear of the creek."

Please let me be right, I prayed.

"How do you know?" he asked me.

"I just talked to him on my radio."

"Well I'm going back up there to be with her."

"That's a good idea," I agreed.

"Okay, she's only about a quarter mile away," he said.

"I'll hurry," I told him. "Oh, uh, sir, is there another road out of here?"

"Nope," he said. "One way in, one way out." Then he turned and galloped away on his horse.

One way in, one way out. Down the washboard logging trail and back across the creek.

Not with this patient.

"Portable 291 to 291."

"This may scratch her up a bit," John said to Joe as he set the blade of the backhoe under the rear bumper of the ambulance.

Joe shrugged. "I can get another bumper."

John gave the thumbs up. "Here goes," he shouted.

"Go ahead, Portable 291," Joe answered.

"Joe, call Orange and see if we can get Pegasus."

"The ambulance is out," he exclaimed. "I'm on my way."

"We're still going to need the helicopter," I told him.

Minutes later, I reached her.

I knelt down and took her hand in mine. "My name is Pat," I said. "I'm sorry it took so long to get here, but we're going to get you to a hospital real soon."

"Thank you," she said. "My neck hurts so bad."

I heard over my portable, "Orange to 291. Pegasus has a ten minute ETA."

"It's going to be okay," I told her.

"You've done a good job keeping her still," I said to her husband.

He nodded and kissed the woman gently on the forehead.

Mine Run's fire department was paged to set up a landing zone. We were less than ten yards from an open field, and the farmer who owned the land was on his way to cut through the barbed wire for us.

I took her pulse and respirations, both rapid. I did a secondary survey, noting facial lacerations, bleeding from the nose, and a contusion with severe swelling on her forehead. Her cervical spine area was tender to the touch, and she had diminished sensation and movement in all four extremities.

Joe reached us in the ambulance just as Pegasus landed.

We put a collar on her neck and started an IV, bandaged her head, rolled her carefully onto the backboard, and carried her to the helicopter.

We stood back and closed our eyes against the wind as Pegasus lifted off the ground, then watched it soar above the trees, heading south.

"She'll be all right," I assured her husband. "She has good feeling and movement in her arms and legs. And she'll have a smooth ride to the trauma center."

He nodded. "Thank you," he said. We shook hands with him and told him good-bye, and he rode away, leading his wife's horse behind him.

Before we were down off the logging trail and back across the creek, Pegasus had landed at the trauma center in Charlottesville.

Emergency room X-rays revealed that Karen had fractured two vertebrae in her upper cervical spine. Rough handling could have severed her spinal cord. She probably would have died.

We wrote a letter to the editor of the *Orange County Review*, thanking the people who had made Karen's rescue possible, the friends and neighbors like John Gentry who came from their homes and their businesses to see what they could do to help.

Julian Wise once said, "Were we to know the merit and value of only going from one street to another to serve a neighbor for the love of God, we should prize it more than gold or silver."

It was an early morning call, for difficulty breathing.

She was sitting on the sofa, leaning forward. Her husband was behind her, rubbing her back.

Her breathing was labored. "Got a knot right here," she told us, holding her fist against her chest.

"Does she have any heart problems?" I asked her husband.

"Just some pain sometimes," he said, continuing to rub her back.

"Does she take any medicine for her heart?"

He shook his head. "No."

"Lung problems?" I asked. "Emphysema? Bronchitis?"

"Emphysema," he nodded.

"Respirations are 36," Joe said. "Her blood pressure is 120 over 60."

Joe put a nasal cannula on her and set it at four liters. I took her arm and felt for a pulse.

No way, I thought to myself. It can't be that rapid. Her heart was racing so fast that I couldn't get an accurate count.

I placed the electrodes on her chest, hooked her up to the monitor, and switched it on.

The normal resting heart rate for an adult is between 60 and 80. A rate over 100 is referred to as sinus tachycardia and can be caused by exercise, pain, fever, and shock. Any treatment is for the underlying cause. Over 150, it's supraventricular tachycardia. And that's dangerous.

Her pulse rate was 240.

Paroxysmal supraventricular tachycardia.

We moved her to the ambulance and I called the hospital. Dr. Heard asked me to transmit an EKG strip. We had the telemetry capabilities to send a strip to the hospital so the doctor could see what we were looking at. I was in the ambulance heading east on Route 3 toward

Fredericksburg, and he was sitting in the telemetry room at Mary Washington Hospital. Together, we were treating the patient.

"Start an IV and then try a carotid sinus massage. Let me know when you're ready to do the massage."

Carotid sinus massage is a procedure that can stimulate the vagal nerve and the parasympathetic nervous system, which can in turn slow the heart.

"Mrs. Cooper, I'm going to lower the head of the gurney a little." I located the carotid arteries, first the right, then the left. Pulses were strong. "Can you face the left, please," I asked.

I moved behind her and picked up the radio. "Okay, I'm ready," I told him when he answered me.

"Let's do it."

Again, I located her right carotid artery. Then I pressed down firmly. I kept my eyes on my watch while I massaged the artery and released the pressure promptly at fifteen seconds. There was no change on the monitor. I asked Joe to check her pulse.

"Still the same," he said.

"Mrs. Cooper, can you turn your head to the right now?"

I repeated the procedure on the left carotid.

Sometimes it works and sometimes it doesn't.

I looked at the monitor. The rate remained steady at 240.

"Medic 291, this is Dr. Heard. You copy?"

I reached for the radio. "We copy," I answered him.

"What's your ETA?" he asked.

I glanced out the window. "Still about twenty."

"Okay, let's try some Verapamil. How much does she weigh?"

"About one-sixty."

"Give her five milligrams IV."

Joe got the med box out of the cabinet. Verapamil was one of our new drugs. I'd seen it given once in the hospital. "Gotta watch this one closely," the nurse had said to me. "The patient could go into cardiac arrest."

I opened the box and found the Verapamil, got a syringe and drew it up, then injected it into the port in the IV.

And I watched.

I picked up the phone and called the hospital. "I've given the Verapamil," I told Dr. Heard.

"Okay, I'll keep my eye on the monitor here."

"So far," I said, "nothing's hap — Whoa, did you see that?"

"I saw it," he said, and I could practically see the smile on his face. She converted.

It was beautiful.

Her pulse rate dropped to 110 and her breathing was easier.

"Honey," she said to me, "the knot's gone now."

When we wheeled her into the emergency room, Dr. Heard was there waiting for us.

"Wasn't that something!" I said when I saw him.

He grinned and nodded. "It really was."

Dr. Heard found us before we left the ER to let us know she was doing well.

"Thank you," I said. "That was really an experience."

He smiled at me. "You'd never given Verapamil before, had you, Pat?"

"How did you guess?"

"Don't let me give you a hard time," he told me. "I love your excitement."

It's hard not to get excited.

We had a call early one morning for a diabetic in insulin shock. He'd gone to bed the night before after taking his insulin, but without having his normal evening snack. His seizure awakened his wife at four-thirty. When we arrived on the scene, his blood sugar was so low, we couldn't even get a reading. He was combative and his breathing was rapid and labored. Holly held him on one side and Jerady on the other while I gave him an injection of glucagon.

Within five minutes, he was sitting up and talking to us. We chatted and laughed en route to the hospital.

It's hard not to get excited.

They were celebrating their fifth anniversary at the restaurant near Lake of the Woods. He ordered prime rib. She decided on the lobster Newburg.

"I haven't had that for a long time," she told him.

We were washing the ambulances when the tones went off, which meant we were right there and could respond in less than a minute.

That was good, because with anaphylactic shock, sometimes that's all the time we have.

When we got to her she could barely breathe because of her allergic reaction to the shellfish. Her face was bright red. Her eyes were almost swollen shut and she had hives all over her abdomen, legs, and back.

The hospital ordered epinephrine and Benadryl. She was gasping for breath when Mara injected the Epi. Minutes later, the hives were gone. She was breathing normally and was ready to order dessert.

We carry twenty-five drugs in our med box. We learn the effects and side effects of each drug, the correct dosage, route of administration and how it's supplied, as well as the indications and contraindications.

We are taught that Narcan will pull a person out of the respiratory depression of a narcotic overdose. Lidocaine wipes out PVCs. Atropine speeds up dangerously slow heart rates. Nitroglycerine abates the pain of angina.

We learn that Verapamil will convert supraventricular tachycardia, that D50 will quickly bring a diabetic out of insulin shock, and that epinephrine will open the airway of a person suffering from a severe allergic reaction.

It's in our textbook.

But when we see the hives diminishing, when we feel a pulse drop from 240 to 110, when we hear intelligible words coming from a patient who moments before didn't know where he was or who he was, there's really only one way to describe it.

It's exciting.

Eight

I saw Wanda Gardner at Mary Washington Hospital yesterday. She is a paid professional paramedic with Spotsylvania County and an unpaid professional with the Culpeper County Volunteer Rescue Squad, and their captain. I've known Wanda for seven years. She's rougher around the edges than I am, but we fight the same battles for quality patient care, and we often fight them together. She is one of the people I'd want with me if I were sick or injured.

"This was one of those days," she said to me, smiling, "that reminds me of why I got into this."

The call was at Spotsylvania Mall. "Unresponsive patient in front of Kitt's Music," the dispatcher reported. Fire personnel from the mall were first on the scene. They found the sixty-three-year-old male conscious but confused, with no radial pulses and an unobtainable blood pressure. Suddenly he went unresponsive again, and this time he stopped breathing. They immediately began ventilations.

"I hooked him up to the monitor when we got there," Wanda told me. "V-tach."

We stood in the middle of the telemetry room just off the nurses' station. "Did you still have a pulse?" I asked her.

"Very weak. I started a line and gave him a hundred of lidocaine and nothing happened. Then the hospital told us to give him five of Valium and then to cardiovert. He was starting to turn blue."

"You ready, Pat?" Norm asked me, leaning around the doorway.

"In just a minute," I told him. I turned back to Wanda. "And?"

Her eyes were shining. "Okay, I cardioverted once and he went asystole and then sinus tach, then back to V-tach. I gave him another seventy-five of lidocaine, then cardioverted again, and *wham*, normal sinus rhythm." She smiled broadly. "He's upstairs in ICU right now, probably having lunch."

Those are the calls that remind us why we got into this. Such calls are rare and we cling to their memories, for they sustain and strengthen us. We relive them in our minds and retell them until we've exhausted our listeners.

We know the odds. If CPR is started on a person in cardiac arrest in less than four minutes and if advanced life support procedures are initiated in less that eight minutes, the survival rate is 43 percent. Add five or six minutes and the survival rate drops to 6 percent. So we know what we're up against.

In 1987, when our fireman Harry had a heart attack out on Route 20 in the middle of an extrication, the doctor told him he was the luckiest man alive.

"Harry," he said, "if you'd had that heart attack at home, you'd be dead."

When he collapsed in the street in his heavy turnout gear, we were right there. And we saved him.

It is five o'clock in the morning. The dispatcher breaks into my sleep with the high-pitched tones and the announcement, "Unresponsive male, not breathing." My mind is pressed into wakefulness. I remember it is Mara's team. I hear them mark en route, Mara and Tom, Judy and Donna and Phil.

"Is CPR in progress?" Mara asks.

The dispatcher tells her, "The caller said no one in the house knows how to do CPR."

The man does not survive.

The Shermans lived across the lake from me. They were both in their sixties, both healthy. They enjoyed golf and looked forward to visits each summer from their five grandchildren. Life was good.

Late one evening, Mr. Sherman began having pain in his chest and left arm. He went into the kitchen and mixed a teaspoon of baking soda into a glass of water and drank it.

Mrs. Sherman looked up at him when he returned to the living room.

"Are you all right, dear?" she asked.

He nodded and burped several times. "Just a little indigestion," he told her. "Baking soda helped." He sat back down and picked up the newspaper.

The pressure in his chest worsened. He repositioned himself in his chair, removed his glasses, and closed his eyes. When he raised a hand to his forehead to help quell the dizziness, he felt the dampness on his face.

"Doris," he said, quite softly, "I don't feel good at all."

She got up quickly from her chair and went to him.

"Is it still your stomach?" she asked, taking his hand.

He nodded weakly. "Yes, my stomach and my chest. It could be the flu," he suggested.

"I think you need to see the doctor, Bert."

"There's no doctor open now," he argued.

"We'll call the rescue squad," she said.

"No," he said, "it's not that serious."

His wife felt it was. He was pale and his skin was very wet. "You look like you're having some trouble breathing."

"A little," he admitted.

"Come on, Bert, I'm taking you to the hospital."

She helped him up and they walked slowly to the door. By the time she got him to the car, she was supporting most of his weight. She fastened his seat belt and got in the driver's seat.

"You rest now," she told him, squeezing his hand. "We'll be there in about twenty minutes." She switched on the heat and listened to the whirring sound of the blowers as they traveled west on Route 3, heading for Culpeper.

They were about hallway there when his heart stopped, but the noise of the heater masked the silence of his dying, and it was not until she pulled up in front of the emergency room and tried to awaken him that she realized he was dead.

We might not have been able to save him.

But we were not given the chance.

Neither was he.

We speak to community gatherings of the early warning signals of a heart attack. We say to them, "if you have chest pain or difficulty breathing or weakness and dizziness, call us!"

The back of our ambulance is, in many ways, like a mobile emergency room. We carry a heart monitor and oxygen and heart-saving, lifesaving drugs.

"A call for cardiac arrest is one of the easiest," Dr. Kravetz told me once. "Procedurally speaking, that is."

He's right. There aren't a lot of decisions to be made. It's all written down in protocol. Just watch the cardiac rhythm and follow the directions.

But it is not just an intellectual effort.

These are lives.

Her car was struck on the driver's side. There was very little damage elsewhere. The driver's teenaged granddaughter, uninjured and screaming, was taken out of the passenger side by passers-by while others removed the driver. A fireman arrived on the scene and started CPR.

"She probably had a heart attack and just drifted in front of the oncoming car," the doctor later explained. There were no visible injuries and her aorta was intact.

We worked on the shoulder of the highway for fifteen minutes. The monitor showed an agonal rhythm, a dying heart. I started an IV and Bill gave a milligram of epinephrine, then one of atropine. We tried a fluid challenge.

We moved her onto a backboard and into the ambulance. We repeated the drugs and tried defibrillation. Then we contacted Mary Washington Hospital and requested permission to stop resuscitation efforts, a Code Gray. It was granted.

The coroner arrived on the scene, and we turned our attention to the grieving child while we waited for other family members to arrive.

This was a life.

Like a pebble tossed into still waters, rippling outward, this life had touched and influenced and loved and been loved.

As we struggle to salvage lives, always in our peripheral vision are the faces of wives, husbands, children, friends. Above the sounds of our own voices, above the sounds of our own fiercely beating hearts, we hear the soft, mournful cries.

We lose too many. Many more than we save, because the odds are often insurmountable.

Dr. David Schenck, our medical adviser, constantly tries to educate his patients regarding preventative medicine. "We are maintained, we are kept alive by an organ the size of our fist," he tells them. "An organ easily damaged by cigarettes, by inactivity, by the T-bone steaks that we eat."

Then he adds, "Combine that with the fact that so few people know CPR, and it's no wonder your win-loss columns are so lopsided."

"So why do you do it?" my friend Susan asks me, struggling to understand.

I tell her about Wanda.

Then I tell her about Mr. Jeffries.

He and his wife had been picking beans from their garden most of the morning. Around eleven he told her he was going in the house to rest. She waved to him and said she'd be in shortly.

He was seventy-two years old with a history of coronary artery disease. He'd never had a heart attack, but he did have episodes of angina from time to time. Resting in the porch swing and taking a nitroglycerine usually relieved the chest pain. But, on this day, it didn't.

She found him slumped over in the swing. She couldn't tell if he was breathing.

The dispatcher requested a three-company response, paging Battlefield, Orange, and Lake of the Woods. We were winding down Route 611 and still four miles away when Battlefield's medic unit arrived on the scene.

They had to pull him away from his wife, who was cradling him in her arms. The dog barked noisily at their feet.

From the Battlefield unit, Frank announced "CPR in progress."

"We're direct," I responded.

The unit from Orange pulled up to the scene just ahead of us. I saw Ed and Danny and Rick. "Just tell us what you need," I yelled to Danny.

"Bring a board and let's get him into our ambulance," he said.

Dick parked our unit and Joe carried the backboard toward the house.

The Battlefield crew had started the IV and were getting ready to give Epi. I watched the monitor. "We've got some idioventricular rhythm here," I said. "Any pulse?"

Danny couldn't find a carotid, but we felt good pulses with the CPR, which meant his circulatory system was intact. His wife stood behind the screen door. Someone, a neighbor, stood with her, his arm gentle on her shoulder. Her hand was pressed hard against her mouth, but I could hear her weeping.

"I can't intubate here," Danny said. "Too little space." We had to move him quickly to be able to ensure an adequate airway. Joe placed the backboard next to him. "Stop CPR," Danny said. We rolled him onto the backboard and rushed him into the ambulance.

We checked for a pulse: still nothing. There was definite rhythm on the monitor, appearing to be idioventricular but perhaps junctional, regular and at a rate of fifty-four beats a minute. "Maybe EMD," I said to Danny. "Let's try a fluid challenge."

We masked en route to Mary Washington Hospital.

While Danny intubated, I prepared the large injections of fluid. We again gave Epi and CPR was continued while I injected the fluid boluses into the IV tubing. "Stop CPR."

The rhythm was V-fib. I charged the paddles and placed them on his chest. "Everybody clear," I said. I pressed the buttons and his body jumped with the 200 joules of electricity.

"Check a pulse."

"No pulse. Still V-fib. Fire again."

"Clear!" And again I defibrillated, this time at 300.

"Check a pulse."

"No pulse. Defibrillate at 360. Clear!"

"No pulse. Continue CPR."

"Epi in. Check a pulse."

"No pulse."

"Clear! Fire!"

"Lidocaine. Bolus and drip."

"Defibrillate at 380."

"Check a pulse."

"No pulse. Continue CPR."

We followed the protocol, the five of us, working as one. Perspiration trickled down Dick's face. He and Rick took turns bagging. Danny's legs were beginning to cramp. Someone cracked a window, and the breeze rushed over us, cooling, cleansing. "ETA?" I called to Joe, but the siren covered my words, and so I glanced out the window for my bearings. "Approaching Eley's Ford Road," I told them. "Twelve minutes."

"Another Epi."

"Stop CPR. Check a pulse."

"No pulse."

"Clear. Defibrillate. Check a pulse."

"I have a pulse!" Danny cried.

"You have a pulse?"

"Yeah, yeah," Danny nodded, his fingers pressed against Mr. Jeffries's neck. "No doubt about it, folks." He smiled broadly. "I have a pulse."

I reached for Mr. Jeffries's hand, closed my eyes, and moved my fingers slowly around the site of the radial artery. And I felt it. "A pulse," I said aloud — but barely above a whisper, as if the sound of my voice would drive it away. "A pulse!" Louder now, a shout.

"Yes!" Frank yelled.

"We did it, guys!"

I looked at the monitor. "He's converted," I told them. "He's in atrial fibrillation."

Five minutes out, we called Mary Washington and told them, "We have a pulse. Our patient is still not breathing on his own, but we have pulses now." They told us, "Good job!"

We looked at each other through misty eyes. We high-fived. We were joyful and disbelieving. We'd beaten the odds.

Mr. Jeffries never made it home. We'd known all along the chance of his returning to his house and his garden were slim.

But that day, in the back of the ambulance, with teams from three different squads working together, we'd performed magic.

Nine

The night I was elected rescue captain, Paul Lewis took me aside.
"Pat," he said, resting his hand on my shoulder and smiling that special smile of his that brightens all our days, "the squad is like a machine. You can work on it all you want but there are always going to be parts that just won't work quite like you want them to.

"And you can't let it get you down."

Paul helps keep us focused by what he says, by what he is. He helps keep us whole. He leads us in prayer at our monthly meetings. He is as kind a man as I have ever met. He has a twin brother named Percy, and the two of them and their wives cook up the best barbecued ribs and chicken I've ever eaten. He saves some of their secret recipe sauce for me and I take it home in a ketchup bottle.

Paul was one of my Grubnelednerts.

He joined our squad in 1971, the year it was formed. "We only had fifteen calls the first year," he said.

"How'd you keep up your skills with so few calls?" I asked him.

He laughed. "Pat, we didn't have any skills."

He was just back from the Vietnam War, and he wanted to join the volunteer squad in a nearby town. "They wouldn't let me in," he told me, "because I was black."

"There was a time about eight years ago," he said, "when I went on a 1050. The guy was really drunk, rolled his truck over, and he's lying in the ditch when we get there. I lean over him to check him out, and he yells, 'You get your black hands off me.'" Paul laughs quietly. "Funny thing was, about halfway to the hospital, he's grabbing on to me and begging, 'Don't let me die. Please don't let me die.'"

Paul shrugs it off and tells me it hasn't been too difficult for him.

It is difficult for me and it is hard for me to say to Paul what I feel. I am angry that this man who could wear a United States Army uniform to do battle in Vietnam could not wear a volunteer rescue squad uniform in some parts of Virginia. I am hurt that he would be scorned by those he reached out to help.

"You know," he said to me, "back in the beginning, it was just scoop and scoot. You gotta do that," he reminded me, "when you don't have any skills." We both laughed. "It was rough. Our first call was a shooting over in Mine Run, a fourteen-year-old boy, first day of hunting season. He fell against his gun. It was a twenty-two, and the bullet went in right here," he said, pointing to his right temple.

"No one should have to begin with a call like that," I said. My first call was for a bee sting.

"Yep, that was my very first one," he nodded. "The bullet didn't seem to go in all that far," he said thoughtfully. "You know, sometimes I wonder if we'd had all the things then that we have now, if we could have saved him.

"Can't spend a lot of time wondering and worrying, though," he said. "Can't do that."

Paul helps keep us focused.

"The only thing consistent about a 1050 is its inconsistencies," my old friend John Beery once told me, and our calls for motor-vehicle accidents over the years have proved him right.

Head-ons can be fatal; or those involved might walk away with minor injuries.

Rollovers aren't so bad unless the occupants are unbelted. We once had a patient suspended by his seat belt in his overturned vehicle. He was smiling at us, upside down, when we got there.

Several years ago, a man lost control of his car and crossed two lanes of traffic before going into a ditch. The car was barely scratched. The man, unbelted, had hit the steering wheel, and en route to the hospital he died from a crushed trachea.

A young woman was traveling down Route 20 when she veered to avoid hitting a deer. Her car catapulted into the woods. We found her where she landed, sitting upright against a tree, the car overturned, the front passenger door open and wedged into the ground between her legs. Her arm was severely broken. That was all. But if the car had gone another twelve inches, she could have been cut in half by the door.

To deal with the various accidents, we arm ourselves with what we know we'll need. Cervical collar and backboard, oxygen on the scene if the patient is trapped and hurt severely, trauma box, IV box. And flexibility. "Don't box yourselves in," Dr. Kravetz tells us. "Don't get your mind so set on what you're going to encounter that once you get there you have to spend time adjusting to the reality."

"Hang loose." The advice comes from the back of the classroom and we all laugh.

"You got it," Dr. Kravetz agrees. "Hang loose."

It was five-thirty on a dark November evening. When the tones went off I thought of Woody. "Day teams should end when it gets dark," he'd grumble, years ago, when Team Three was Jean and Buzzy and Woody and me.

Dark or not, I still had thirty minutes left of my twelve-hour shift. It was a wreck on 611, a serpentine country road. "Vehicle overturned," the dispatcher told us. Paul and Barbara and Joe and I started out on the first ambulance. Bill and Donna and Dick brought the second one.

The accident was in the mutual-aid territory we share with Battlefield. I heard Ray's voice, marking their medic unit on the scene. Moments later, he called the dispatcher and requested Pegasus, the Medivac helicopter from University of Virginia Hospital's Trauma Center.

"Pegasus is available with a fifteen minute ETA," the dispatcher informed him.

"Incoming instructions?" I asked Ray when we turned off Route 20 and onto 611.

"Pull up behind us," Ray said. "Your patient's at the car."

Spotlights from the engine and crash truck transformed darkness to light. We pulled up behind Medic 210. I glanced inside as I moved quickly to the overturned car. "Were they doing CPR?" I asked Barbara, beside me.

"I didn't look," she said, her eyes fixed on the car in the field before us. "Pat, those people are talking to someone under the car."

It was a ten-year-old boy.

He had been thrown from the vehicle and was now lodged under it.

I stretched out on the ground and felt the cold earth beneath me. Someone was holding a light, and I could see the child. He was lying on his back. His eyes were open but unfocused. I worked my way a little closer to him and I reached out for his hand.

"Can you feel me holding your hand?" I asked him.

"Yes," he said softly. He began to cry.

I held tightly to his hand. "What's your name?"

"Mark," he said. "My head hurts," he cried, "and my arm."

The avulsion on his head was so deep his skull was exposed. His upper arm was grossly deformed. There was a small laceration where the bone, broken and splintered, had split the skin.

"Can you reach his head?" I asked Barbara, and together we repositioned the flap of skin and applied a bandage to it.

"Hi, Mark," she said to him, her voice soft and comforting. "My name's Barbara."

"I think he's free," I said to her. I ran my hands down both his legs and didn't feel anything snaring, pinning him under the car. "Tell Joe to get a backboard. I think we can slide him out."

"Where's my mama?" he asked me.

"She's in another ambulance," I explained. "Someone else is taking care of her." It was the truth.

He started to cry again. "Is she okay?"

"I haven't seen her, darling, but I'm sure they are taking real good care of her."

"When they took her away, her eyes were closed."

Joe came up with the backboard.

"Mark," I told the boy, "we're going to put a big white collar on you. It won't hurt," I assured him. "Then we're going to get you out."

We moved him slowly onto the backboard. I held his arm, trying to stabilize it. Once he was free of the car, we moved him quickly to the ambulance.

"Pat — " Ray said. He was standing at the rear of the ambulance. " — you want Pegasus for the boy?"

"Yes," said. "Multiple trauma. I thought you'd already called," "I told him.

He nodded. "I did. They'll be on the ground in about two minutes."

"Good."

"Can I talk to you a minute?" he asked.

I glanced at Mark. Barbara and Paul were doing the assessment. Bill was setting up a line of Ringers.

"Be right back," I said to them and stepped off the ambulance.

Ray was waiting for me.

"I'd called the helicopter for his mother but we lost her," he said. "We'd been doing CPR since we got her out of the car. UVA said we could call it."

I had told Mark that the others were taking good care of her. I hadn't lied.

Above us, Pegasus circled. I closed my eyes against the sudden gusts of wind.

I stood aside, there if they needed me, but away from Mark's questions. I watched Barbara holding tightly to his hand when Bill started the IV. They'd put the MAST trousers on him and splinted his arm and applied additional bandages to his head. Barbara and Joe could easily answer the questions posed by the Pegasus crew — time trapped, any loss of consciousness, how much bleeding.

They could also answer Mark's questions with greater ease. Because they didn't know the truth.

But when the helicopter lifted off, I told them. Barbara, as I knew she would, cried. I stood with her beside me, with my arm around her as we watched Pegasus disappear into the night sky.

In the summer of 1989, the summer Uncle Roy died, Jennifer had her tonsils taken out. As my parents had promised me on the eve of my tonsillectomy, so did I promise her — all the ice cream she wanted.

Her father, David, met us at the hospital the next morning.

"Dr. Kravetz is the anesthetist," I told him. "At least I feel confident about that."

"It's a simple procedure," David said. "I don't know why you're worried."

We were with her while she was prepped. Dr. Kravetz told Jennifer jokes as he started the IV on her, and she didn't even flinch.

"Don't you tell her the ones you tell us in class," I said. "She's way too young."

He winked at her. "Just wait until we get rid of your mother."

We stayed until they were ready to take her into the operating room. I kissed her cheek softly, "I love you," I told her.

"Love you, too, Mom," she said.

I waved good-bye. "See you soon."

"About forty-five minutes," Dr. Kravetz said. "We'll see you in recovery."

"You want a Coke or something?" David asked me.

I glanced at my watch. "Is the cafeteria okay?" I asked, not wanting to leave the hospital.

"That's fine."

I felt secure there, with Jennifer two floors above me. There was security for me, too, just having her in Mary Washington Hospital. I knew the floors, the halls. She was born there. I'd trained there. I knew nurses and doctors and pharmacists and every nook and cranny of the emergency room.

"You want something to eat?" he asked me.

"No, thank you," I said.

I looked across at him. It had been more than three years since he'd left, and yet there was much about him, about us, that I still missed.

"The last time we were here with her was a lot more pleasant," I said.

"Yes," he smiled, and just for a moment, our eyes met.

I finished my coffee. "You ready to go back?" I asked him.

"Yeah," he said. "I guess it's time."

"Forty-five minutes on the nose," he said as we approached the entrance to the operating suite. "I guess this is where they'll come out. You want to go into the waiting room and sit down?"

"No," I told him. "I'll wait here."

Twenty minutes later we were still waiting. It was another twenty minutes before Dr. Kravetz came through the door.

He walked up to me. "Well," he said, "there's been a problem."

"There's been a problem?" I echoed his words. "What kind of problem?"

This was a simple tonsillectomy.

"Let's go sit down," he said, taking my arm.

David and I sat on the sofa in the waiting room. Dr. Kravetz sat in a chair across from us. "Some people," he began, "have a very low level of pseudocholinesterase. Big word, I know. And an important enzyme in that when patients have a general anesthetic, it's the pseudocholinesterase that enables them to start breathing on their own again."

This was my teacher. I'd been listening to his medical explanations for five years. He was supposed to be standing in front of the class-room telling me how to take care of other people's emergencies.

But he was explaining to me why my daughter wasn't breathing.

He took my hand when I began to cry. "This happens sometimes," he said. "Pat, she's going to be okay."

"When?" I asked.

"Probably a couple of hours."

A lifetime.

"Why didn't you know this?" David asked. "I thought you did a lot of blood work."

"We did, but unfortunately the way you discover a person has a lack of pseudocholinesterase is when they don't start breathing on their own after the anesthesia starts to wear off. That is the test.

"I'll be back every twenty minutes. Okay?" He said, squeezing my hand. "To let yon know how she's doing."

"How is she breathing now?" I asked.

"We have her sedated and on a ventilator," he said.

He left then, but, true to his word, he came back every twenty min-utes. David and I sat in the room, alone. Once, he put his hand on mine. I need more, I screamed at him, silently. This is our daughter. Just put your arms around me. Not for forever, just for now.

Four hours and fifteen minutes later, they took her off the ventila-tor. She was breathing on her own. David and I walked with her as they rolled her to her room. She had IVs in both arms and she was still sedated.

We stayed with her until she woke up. Her throat hurt too much to talk. We kissed her and told her how much we loved her.

"Stay with us tonight," I asked David.

But he had to go.

I spent the night beside her, so near that I could hold her hand while she slept. I dozed a little, always lightly, and each time I awoke I would whisper to her, "I love you."

Jennifer was released from the hospital the next day. Three weeks later, we packed up for our traditional summer trip to Topsail Island,

North Carolina. "We can't forget my telescope," Jennifer reminded me. "Nana says there's going to be an eclipse." We rented a house on the beach and filled it with music and laughter and the smell of fish cooking.

David, Jr., was twenty that year, and Matt eighteen; my sons, big and boisterous and tender and loving.

Jennifer and Jenny entered a sand castle-building contest and won first place. "It was the crabs crossing the drawbridge that won it," Jenny beamed.

"It was a stroke of genius," my father said, winking at my mother.

"I know," Jennifer said. "It was Nana's idea."

"Oh, but you girls lined them up perfectly," she said, smiling and hugging them both.

Jenny is six weeks older than Jennifer. They've been best friends since they were born. "You know," I tell Jenny, "the first time I held you in my arms, Jennifer kicked you. But you've been best friends ever since."

Each day, we'd all search for shark's teeth in the sand. We'd drag our floats into the ocean and ride the tides back to shore. We fished for flounder and blue. We'd walk to the end of the island early in the morning and then again at sunset, all of us together.

On Wednesday morning we got the telescope out and set it up on the porch.

"We're really lucky," David told us. "It said in the paper that the eclipse is only going to be visible in the eastern part of the United States. It's going to begin at sunset right after the moon rises. And," he continued, "for your added pleasure, ladies and gentlemen, you will also be able to see meteors from the Perseid meteor shower."

We sat in a row on the porch that night like moviegoers anxious for the feature to start. We watched the moon surface on the distant horizon, watched it climb into the night sky, and fixed it in our sights while we sang, "I see the moon and the moon sees me, down through the leaves of the old oak tree, God bless the moon and God bless me and God bless the one I love."

At nine-thirty, the earth's shadow began to slowly cross the moon. We took turns gazing through the telescope. We "oohed" and "aahed" and giggled with excitement. By eleven, the eclipse was complete, and we walked down from the porch onto the beach and spread blankets on the sand and lay down and gazed into the heavens.

"I'm glad you all are my family," I said above the roar of the ocean to the people around me as we watched in wonder the meteors streak across the sky.

There are certain moments in our lives that are so full, so perfect, so glorious, that we sense our unworthiness for such happiness and we hold our breath, in silence, in absolute stillness, afraid to even move far fear those moments will require payback.

Such was that moment.

Ten

Dr. Kravetz told us a story once about a patient who was in supraventricular tachycardia with a pulse rate of 180. The doctors had tried Verapamil to lower the rate, but it hadn't worked. They decided to cardiovert.

"She was sitting up and talking to us," he said. "So I was explaining to her what the procedure would be like, a little shock. I told her I was going to give her a mild sedative before we attempted cardioversion. And — " he said, his eyes widening — "at that point I reached out and took her hand in mine.

"And she converted on her own!"

This is a story Bernie Siegel would cherish.

Bernie Siegel is a surgeon and the author of *Love, Medicine and Miracles*. He is a true believer in the holistic theory that "whole entities have an existence other than the mere sum of their parts"; as it relates to medicine, in "care of the entire patient in all aspects."

I once heard him speak. Persuasive and dynamic, he would make the most cynical believe in the magic of touch. His lectures contain stories of the healing power of love. He tells of an interesting study of women in labor. Of those women who had someone with them for support, only seven percent asked for an epidural anesthesia. Of the women who had no one with them but were aware of others in the room, twenty-two percent requested anesthesia. Of the women who were left all alone, fifty-five percent asked for an epidural.

Roy was in congestive heart failure. We'd frequently taken him to Mary Washington Hospital. Several months ago he'd hesitated in calling us, and we almost lost him. There had been fluid in his lungs and he could barely breathe. His blood pressure was severely elevated. We put him on high-flow oxygen and administered morphine and Lasix, a diuretic. Soon, his BP began to come down, and he was breathing easier.

We saved his life.

I saw him several weeks later. Each time he tried to talk, his eyes filled with tears. "I'm sorry," he said, reaching for his handkerchief.

I knew it was difficult for him to talk about the fact that he had come so close to dying. "It's all right," I told him. "That's what we're here for." The doctors had told him he probably would not be alive if we had not treated him quickly and aggressively.

He took a deep breath. "I just want to thank you."

"I understand," I said.

"Whoever it was who had their hand on my shoulder on the way to the hospital," he said, again wiping away the tears, "I'll never forget it. It got me through."

That was what he remembered.

And he attributed his survival to the hand on his shoulder.

Who's to say he was wrong?

Sally's father was a doctor. "He always told me to make sure I gave ten percent back to life," she remembers, smiling. "And he wasn't talking about money," she says. "He was talking about service."

I met Sally when Jennifer and Emily, Sally's daughter, were in nursery school together. Later, she and I served together as Brownie leaders. I was on the squad, and it was then that I started recruiting her.

"You kept pushing me into what I was destined to become," she said to me on her first night in EMT class.

"I know," I said, giving her a hug. "We all need a push from time to time."

In 1958, when she was three years old, Sally's father suffered a massive heart attack. "We'd gone to our farm in Middletown for the day," she said. "The ambulance took him all the way back to Arlington. Of course, you could hardly call it an ambulance. There was nothing inside but the gurney, no oxygen, nothing. And both attendants rode up front. Knowing what I know now, it's hard to believe he made it. And we had him with us for another thirty-one years.

"I was frightened but I was fascinated, too," she admitted. "Maybe that's where it all began," she said, smiling.

We had just returned from a call for a minor 1050 and were finishing the paperwork when the pickup truck tore into the parking lot. The driver was lying on the horn.

I ran to the passenger side and opened the door. The young man inside had his hands over his face. Blood was trickling down between his fingers.

"What happened?" I asked the driver.

"We were working on the new sewer line," he said, breathing hard. "He was in the ditch checking the pressure and a piece blew off in his face. Knocked him over backwards. His head's all torn up."

"Sally, put a collar on him and let's get him out of here," I said. Joe and Scott were getting the backboard on the gurney.

"Let me see," I said to the man.

He moved his fingers slightly away, and I could see the deep gash in his forehead, above his right eye. The bleeding had slowed, but the swelling was intense. His eye was almost swollen shut.

"Okay, Larry," the man next to him said. "You're going to be okay."

Sally had put the cervical collar on him and was bandaging his head. "He's right, Larry," she told him. "You're going to be okay."

We moved him onto the gurney and lifted him onto the ambulance. The first set of vitals were good. I started an IV of Ringers en route to Mary Washington.

"Let's get another blood pressure," I said to Joe.

Sally was holding ice packs against Larry's bandaged forehead. We'd raised the backboard slightly to elevate his head.

"His blood pressure is up a little," he said. "Pulse has slowed, too." Signs of closed head injury.

I cut the flow rate back on the IV.

"Talk to him, Sally," I said. "Let's get a level of consciousness. Then we'll call the hospital." We were fifteen minutes out.

"Larry," she said. "How's your head feel now?"

He tried to turn his head to face her but the collar and head immobilizer prevented him from moving.

It started with a moan and quickly escalated to a scream. He reached out for Sally. Fearing he'd pull the IV out, I took hold of his arm and forced his wrist into a restraint.

"Twenty-five, thirty-five, no, no, God, no," he yelled, over and over. Sally was leaning across his chest now, trying to restrain him. Joe was holding his left arm down while I tried to work that wrist into a restraint. "What's he saying?" I asked Joe.

"He must have known it was going to blow by watching the pressure rise," Joe explained.

"God, no, thirty-five, thirty-five," he screamed.

I called up to Scott, "Expedite!"

"Have you all got him?" I asked Joe and Sally. "I've got to call the hospital."

"I think so," Sally said.

I stood up and reached for the phone. "Medic 292 to Mary Washington Hospital."

They answered and Larry screamed. He was kicking now. I gave the hospital personnel the information quickly, hoping they could hear me. There was no way I could hear them.

"You're going to have to get his legs," Joe told me. "I can't move from here." It was taking both of them to hold his chest and his arms, even with restraints. He kept arching his back, trying to throw them off.

I sat on his ankles, but he pulled his feet through my legs. I moved up and sat on his knees. He could still lift me.

I glanced out the window. "We're a block away," I told them. "Hold on."

At the hospital, Scott had to go inside and get extra help while we held our positions on Larry.

They sedated him, intubated him, and flew him by Med-star to the Washington Trauma Center. The doctors told us later that although the injury was bad, he would suffer no permanent damage. "It was the psychological trauma that was so severe," they said. "Knowing what was coming. It scared the hell out of him."

"Scared the hell out of us, too," I admitted.

"I thought maybe it was me," Sally said to us later.

"What was you?" I asked her.

"Well, he didn't scream until he looked at me."

Sally's father died in 1989 of a very rare and inoperable cancer of the gall bladder. The next year, she joined the rescue squad.

"I know he knows what I'm doing," she told me one day after a very difficult call. "I just wish he could be here."

I had just dropped the spaghetti into the boiling water when the tones went off.

"Attention Lake of the Woods Rescue Squad members, you have a call on Westover Parkway for an infant hung on a chain."

Jennifer looked up from her science book. "What did he say?"

I looked at her. "Infant hung on a chain?"

"How could an infant get hung on a chain?" she asked me.

I shrugged. "I don't know. Maybe that's not what they said."

"I'll watch the spaghetti," she offered. "You go see."

I wasn't on duty and the location of the call wasn't near our house. But it was a baby.

"Okay," I said. "I won't be long. The spaghetti will be done in five minutes. Don't forget."

"I won't forget, Mom."

"I love you," I said, kissing the top of her head.

"Love you, too."

I heard the ambulance mark en route as I got in my car. I heard Holly's voice. "What was the nature of the call?" she asked, and I listened closely.

"An infant hung on a chain," he repeated.

"A chain?" she asked again.

"That's what they said. A chain."

I turned onto Lakeview with terrible images in my mind. Was it a swag chain on a light? If so, how would an infant get hung on that? Could it have been a chain-link fence? That made a little more sense, but not much more. I glanced in my rearview mirror and saw Bill behind me. Behind him was Joe.

"Rescue 292 is on the scene," Holly said.

I wondered if they'd need a cardiac technician. I pushed on the accelerator and saw Bill move closer behind me. He was surely wondering the same thing.

An infant hung on a chain. A toy, I thought, perhaps. But what kind of toy would have a chain on it that would hang an infant? I was three blocks away.

"Rescue 292 to LOW," Holly said. "Everything is fine here." She sounded amused. "You can 1022 any other responding units."

"Ten-four," the LOW dispatcher acknowledged.

I was too close to turn around. And too curious. I started to pull in front of the house but these was no room. Aside from the ambulance crew, Norm was there, and Sally and Kirk. Bill and Joe were still behind me, and Bobby and Art were coming in from the other end of the street. And Wes had run over from his house to save the "infant hung on a chain."

I parked several houses away, got out of my car, and walked toward the house. Holly was just coming out, and she was still laughing.

The new parents had just bathed their baby. They had placed her on the changing table to dry her off and powder her, and her foot had gotten caught momentarily in the side support.

They had been upset when they called security. "Our baby was hung on the changing table," they said, hurriedly. "We'd like someone to look at her foot."

New parents, new dispatcher. "Infant hung on a chain."

"Jennifer," I said when I walked in the door, "you're not going to believe this."

We move quickly for children.

"Possible drowning at Ramsey Beach," the dispatcher told us. "Eleven-year-old."

We do not have to be told to expedite.

He'd gone into the lake shortly after eating lunch and tried to follow the older boys into the deeper water. It was then that he got the stomach cramp. He tried to yell but couldn't, then held his arm up to signal to anyone who might be looking.

Fortunately, his mother was.

"I think something's wrong with Tommy," she said to her daughter.

"Why?" the child asked, looking up.

At that moment, he went under.

The mother screamed and then rushed toward the water. Someone ran to a nearby house and called for help.

Jerady and Darren were already there when we arrived. And Sally.

"His mother pulled him out of the water," Sally told me, as we knelt beside the boy. His eyes were closed but he was breathing. I found his pulse easily. It was strong and regular. "The woman over there said she did some ventilations on him," Sally continued. "He was breathing when I got here. Boy, what a relief!"

We lifted him onto the gurney and moved him to the ambulance. He was listless and coughing some, and we were afraid he'd aspirated water.

He opened his eyes and looked around.

"My name's Pat," I told him. "And this is Barbara. And Tom and Norm."

"We're going to take good care of you," Barbara said, taking his hand in hers.

"That's your assignment," I said to her, seeing that she had already begun to ease his fears.

"Good," she smiled. "It's my favorite job."

She talked to him while I started the IV and he barely flinched.

His breathing remained rapid, but his EKG and his other vitals looked good. Barbara kissed him good-bye when we left him at Culpeper Memorial Hospital. They would keep him overnight for observation and the next day, he would be back at the beach.

"Darn," Barbara said, on our trip back. "We forgot to give him a teddy bear."

"He's probably a little old for a stuffed animal," Tom said. "Don't you think?"

I shook my head. "You never get too old."

We have an odd assortment of dolls and stuffed animals. Most are donations. The bears are my favorites. Tyler loved his dragon. But Mr. Fagan had his eye on the donkey.

"Your hands are mighty cold, little lady," he said to me as I was putting the patches on his chest. I hooked him up to the cardiac monitor.

"I'm sorry, Mr. Fagan," I told him. "We should have hand warmers in here, shouldn't we?"

"Just stick 'em in your armpits," he suggested. "That'll work."

His EKG showed atrial fibrillation.

"Squeeze my hands, Mr. Fagan," I asked him. His right hand was strong, but there was very little pressure from the left one. I noted it on the call sheet.

"I'm going to take your blood pressure," Joe said. "It's going to get a little snug on your arm."

"Are your hands cold, too?" he asked.

"Probably," Joe answered him. "It's pretty chilly out today."

Mr. Fagan had always been healthy and, at seventy-two, was very independent. But, earlier, on this day, his daughter had stopped by to see him and found him unable to move his left side.

"190 over 120," Joe said.

Too high.

Mr. Fagan looked around him. He watched the electrical tracing of his heart bob up and down across the monitor. "Look okay?" he asked, too casually, seemingly uninterested. But I knew better.

"It looks pretty good," I told him. "It's a little irregular. You can see that, but your pulse at both your wrists is good and strong, and that's good."

He seemed to be satisfied with my answer and nodded his approval.

I asked Joe to call the hospital and then turned back to Mr. Fagan.

"I'm going to start an IV on you now," I said, "and you're going to feel a little needle stick."

He was looking at the cabinet where we keep the stuffed animals.

"Are your hands any warmer?" he asked me.

"They are," I told him. "Feel." And I rested my hand on his arm.

"Yeah, that's better. What's that thing looking down at me?"

I glanced at him and then in the direction where he was looking.

I smiled. "Looks like a donkey to me," I said. "Hold really still now." I started the line and taped it.

"The hospital says to give a nitro for the blood pressure," Joe said, reaching for the med box.

"I think you got so many of those little things up there that donkey's 'bout to fall out," Mr. Fagan said.

I stood up and looked in the cabinet. "You're right," I told him. "It is crowded in there." I took the donkey out. It was fluffy and brown with big floppy ears. "Since he's had his eye on you, how about you take him?" I said.

"Might as well," he said gruffly.

I put it in his lap. "There you go," I said.

Joe handed me the small bottle of nitroglycerine.

"Open wide. This goes under your tongue," I told him, placing the small pill there. "Okay, just let it dissolve. You'll probably get a headache but it won't last long. And this will help get your blood pressure down."

He picked up the donkey and placed it in the crook of his left arm.

"I used to have a donkey that looked like this one," he said, stroking its ears. "Long time ago."

"Well, then, you're the perfect owner for him," I said.

Five minutes later, Joe took another blood pressure. This time it was 160 over 90.

"You're looking good, Mr. Fagan," I told him.

"Feeling pretty good, too," he said.

When we pulled up to the hospital loading dock he asked me if we wanted the donkey back.

"No," I told him. "He belongs to you."

We wheeled him into the emergency room. After we'd exchanged our IV and drug boxes and changed the sheets on the gurney, we stopped to say good-bye. He'd fallen asleep on the stretcher with the donkey still in his arms.

Eleven

The phone rang at 7:45.
It was a Monday morning in September 1989.

"Honey," my mother began. It was a good connection.
She sounded so close, her words clear and sharp. "Daddy's had a heart attack."
Too clear. Too sharp. No mistake in what she'd said. "How bad is it?" I asked, and I began to cry. "It's bad," she told me. She was crying now. "I'll be there by noon," I said. "Tell him I love him."

Matt was a student at Germanna Community College and Jennifer was a seventh grader, in her first year at Prospect Heights Middle School. David was across the mountain, a junior at James Madison University.
I had phone calls and arrangements to make.

It is a three-and-a-half-hour drive from Wilderness to Salem. I listened to the radio most of the way but there were dead spots around Louisa County and then again between Staunton and Lexington. So I had too much time to think.
Years ago, when I decided to become a cardiac technician, I was aware that this moment could come, an early morning phone call, a heart attack. I somehow felt that my intellectual knowledge would prepare me. I'd know what to look for and I'd know what questions to ask the doctor. But the scenarios in my mind were always hypothetical. And this road passing beneath me was real. And nothing can ever really soften the blow.
My father's best friend was a man named Givens Gardner. He was a tall, slender man with eyes of azure blue, and always whistling. He was

a fisherman, like Daddy. They could fish together for hours and not talk because they were friends and there was no unease in their silences. His wife, Nelle Oakey, taught elementary school with my mother. She was my third-grade teacher at North Cross School, and aside from my parents and grandparents, they were the best, most decent people I ever knew. During my senior year in college, Givens Gardner was diagnosed with cancer. The carcinoma was in the late stages when the doctors found it. My parents would go to the hospital each evening. In the middle of Givens's second week in the hospital, Daddy got a phone call and the news that his brother, Cecil, had suffered a stroke. "I'm on my way," he told my aunt in Phoenix. To Givens, he said, "I'll be back in less than a week." His brother died before he got to Arizona; his friend died before he came home. Life is not fair.

I wondered, would my father be alive when I got to Salem?

He taught me how to ride a bike and he taught me how to drive and how to put a worm on a hook and how to take a catfish off. He taught me that the black man who cleaned the bathrooms at the First Methodist Church was just as important as the minister. He tried to teach me algebra.

He said, "Always stand up when the flag goes by," and I always do. He said things to me like "Never judge a man until you've walked in his shoes" and "I cried because I had no shoes until I saw a man who had no feet." He was the smartest man I ever knew. And the funniest. I wondered, would he be alive when I got to Salem?

"He's about the same," my mother told me. We sat together in the Cardiac Care lounge of Lewis Gale Hospital. There is no joy in that room, and any good news is always relative.

"We can go back in at two," she said. "But only for about ten minutes." It was the first chance we'd had to talk since her phone call that morning. I had driven straight to the hospital and seen him briefly. The nitro drip made him nauseous and the Phenergan made him drowsy. I could do little more than hold his hand and tell him I loved him.

"They say they really won't know for about twenty-four hours how much damage there is," my mother said, and I knew they were preparing her for the reality of cardiogenic shock or congestive heart failure.

"I heard him get up," she said. "He went into the kitchen and got a bowl of cereal. I heard the spoon against the bowl," she said, smiling.

"Then I must have dozed off. I could see the light was still on in the kitchen when I woke up. And I heard him walking toward the bedroom.

"When he reached the door, he just stood there, in the dark. I switched on the light above our bed and I saw his face. He was so pale. He said, 'Edna, you'd better can the rescue squad. I think I'm having a heart attack.'"

"What did they do when they got there?" I asked her.

"Well, when I called 911, the woman said it would be about twenty minutes before she could get an ambulance, so I drove him here."

"You drove him?" I said, remembering the Shermans.

"The woman asked how close we were to the hospital," she explained. "I just didn't want to wait."

"Oh, Mama, I know," I told her, taking her hand in mine. She looked so frail, so anxious. Suddenly, I felt as if I were interrogating her. "You want some coffee?" I asked.

"No, I don't think so." She was staring out into the hallway. "I wish the doctor would come."

In the background, Oprah droned on. A peach-jacketed hospital volunteer poured water into the coffee urn. "Wait until the red light comes on," she said.

Mama glanced at her watch.

"I wonder if Daddy is counting the seconds like we are."

She smiled at me. "I'm so glad you're here," she said.

"So am I," I told her.

I couldn't bear the thought of her being alone.

"You know," I said to her. "I've never seen you paint." Her paintings are spectacular, oil paintings of sea shells, old barns, and farmer's markets.

"You have four of them hanging in your house," she said.

"I have your paintings," I explained. "But I've never watched you while you were painting a picture. I'd like to do that sometime."

"All right," she said. "I'd like that too."

What else had I left undone?

Because there is always tomorrow.

At five o'clock we entered the Cardiac Care Unit. Daddy was still asleep. His chart hung on a clip by the door. I took it down and looked at it. "Should you do that?" my mother asked.

"It's all right," I assured her.

My father stirred in his sleep. She raised her finger to her lips, "Shhh," she whispered.

On his chart I saw the electrocardiogram printout from the night before, the severe ST elevation, the PVCs reflecting the irritability of his heart. The blood gases, enzymes, medications . . . lidocaine, morphine, Stepto. . . .

I walked quietly out to the nurses' station. "Excuse me," I said to the nurse at the desk.

"Yes?" she answered.

"I am Mr. Follmar's daughter," I told her. "My mother wants to know if the doctor will be in to see him this afternoon."

"He was here this morning," she said.

"Yes, but she missed him then and she'd like to see him sometime today. She is very worried."

"I'll see if I can reach him," she told me.

I felt so helpless. I could read his electrocardiogram but I couldn't find a doctor. I could learn more about the condition of a stranger at Mary Washington Hospital than I could here about my own father.

I walked back into his room. His eyes were open and Mama was leaning close to him, talking.

"Hi, Doc," he said when he saw me.

I leaned across the lines leading to the monitor and the IV and kissed him gently on the cheek. "Hi, Daddy. How are you feeling?"

"Better," he said. But he looked pale, and his voice was very weak.

"Our time's almost up," Mama said.

"But Doc just got here," he said.

"I'm not far away," I told him. "Just down the hall. And we'll be back before you know it."

"Okay," he said and closed his eyes again.

The doctor came in later that afternoon. He looked at the results of the latest blood tests and electrocardiogram. Then he listened to Daddy's chest with his stethoscope. "Al," he said, and his voice was soft and kind, "have you had any more pain today?"

"No," he said. "Don't want any more, either." Later, the doctor told me that Daddy's condition was critical.

The next day, Matt and Jennifer drove over the mountain and picked up David, and the three of them came to Salem. We could still only go in two at a time. Jennifer and I went in first, then Matt and David.

She stood at the foot of his bed. "Hi, Papa," she said softly. Her eyes followed the IV tubing snaking down from the bottles and going to both his arms. The cardiac monitor beeped. Tears welled in her eyes.

"Hi, Rosebud." His name for her since she was a baby. "Her mouth looks like a rosebud," he had said when he first saw her. She was only a day old, pink and wrinkled and beautiful. "Did you bring your flute?" he asked her.

She laughed then. And that was good. "No, Papa," she said. "But I will next time."

She looked at me as if perhaps she'd said something wrong. I smiled at her. I wanted her to know that I believed there would be a next time, too. He would hear her play her flute again. She moved closer to him and pressed her hand against his.

"Are you okay, Papa?" she asked.

"I will be, sweetheart," he said. "I will be."

He was in the hospital for three weeks and while he was there, he suffered two more heart attacks. His heart was so badly damaged, he was not a viable candidate for bypass surgery.

Twice, we made hurried trips to his bedside. On a quiet Sunday afternoon in early October, my father and my sons got to say to each other all the things that men so rarely get to say, quiet expressions of love, poignant narratives of happy memories, and soft, soft whispers of goodbye.

He wrote us this poem. He called it "Papa's Pride."

> Edna makes the canvas glow
> Oakey is our prize to show
> Patricia makes the stanzas grow
> Rosebud gets the flute to sing
> Dave-Boy can do most anything
> Matt-Jon has the world in tow
> Papa's pride is a bottomless spring.

I called Bob Kravetz late that night. "How can he live," I asked him, "if his heart is that bad?"

"Collateral circulation," he explained. "The heart is taking care of itself. The vessels sprout and expand. It can work, Pat," he said, his voice calm and reassuring.

"I hope so," I told him.

Dr. Kravetz was right. It did work. It worked for almost three years.

Twelve

Dr. Schenck is our family physician. He was born in Pine Bluff, Arkansas, and grew up in McComb, Mississippi, and he readily admits he was destined to become a rural doctor. At thirty-eight, he is tall and lanky and quiet spoken. I've never seen him in a white coat. His patients love him and reward him with chocolate cakes and home-made bread and fresh venison in hunting season.

He told me once that he tried to treat all patients as if they were his relatives, his parents, spouse, children, brother, or sister. "That way," he said, "I give them my best."

I thought a lot about that during the weeks my father was in the hospital as I observed those who cared for him. I watched closely for nuances and listened to the messages in their words and in their silences. It soon became clear to me who shared Dr. Schenck's philosophy and who did not.

When I returned to Wilderness, I brought with me an added dimension to my care and a greater understanding of our responsibility. It is always easier and safer to distance ourselves, to fix our positions on the outside, looking in.

We can't do that, of course. Instead, we must look deeper into our patient's eyes, allowing our hands to linger on theirs after the pulse count, always giving proof with our actions what we profess with our words, "We're going to take good care of you."

I knelt on the floor in front of him. His skin was hot and his eyes listless, feverish.

"He can't eat," his wife told me. She rubbed her hands together, nervous gestures. Her fingers were knotted with arthritis. "Our children don't live close by and I can't get him to the doctor."

He was a large man. He sat erect in his chair.

"Tell me what's wrong, Mr. Morris," I asked him. The dispatcher had told us only, "Eighty-one-year-old male. Unknown illness."

"Can't keep nothing down," he said. "For two days." He glanced at his wife, then looked back toward me. "Never been in an ambulance before."

I smiled at him. "It's not so bad," I told him. "We'll try to be good company for you."

We helped him up from his chair and walked him out to the ambulance. Dick helped Mrs. Morris into the front passenger seat and tightened the seat belt for her. Doris and I rode in the back with Mr. Morris.

His pulse and respirations were somewhat rapid, but that's to be expected with a fever. His blood pressure was good and he wasn't in any pain.

"Have you had a cough?" I asked. "Or any type of infection?"

"No, no cough," he said. "Do you think I'm very sick?"

"No," I told him. "I don't think so."

Silently, I ruled out sepsis. I also didn't mink it was pneumonia. His lung sounds were clear and he had no pain or difficulty breathing. Probably the flu, but that can be fatal for the very young and the very old. And the dehydration can lead to hypovolemic shock.

I kept my hand on his arm during the twenty-minute trip. We didn't talk much, but as his fear diminished, he began to relax. In the hospital, we moved him from the gurney to the stretcher, then gave our report to the nurse.

I pulled up a chair next to the stretcher so his wife could sit next to him.

"Thank you," he said to us as we turned to go. "You were right." He smiled. "That ambulance wasn't so bad."

Dick returned his smile. "We were hoping you'd say that."

We left them, our patient and his wife. She sat beside him, holding his large hand in her twisted one.

They were someone's parents.

They could have been mine.

He was dead when we got there. Face-up on the sofa, full of cocaine, clad only in his underwear, in a shack down at the bottom of a dead-end road. Police cruisers parked in the dirt driveway, blue lights spinning.

"Makes me sick," the large-bellied deputy muttered. Flies swarmed around the dead man, some lighting on his face, walking over his eyelids. Outside, a woman screamed.

"Can you take him to the morgue?" the deputy asked me.

I nodded. "How old do you think he was?" I asked.

"Oh, eighteen, twenty, I guess," he said. "God, just look at this place."

There wasn't much to look at, though — two rooms, a sofa and TV, a refrigerator, rotted floors, walls full of holes, rat feces.

Joe and I stepped down to the front yard, less a yard than an extension of the dirt drive. A crowd had gathered, women holding babies, older dark-eyed children, sullen men, all watching us.

"Norm," I said, "we've got to take him to the morgue."

He and Joe pulled the gurney off the ambulance. I stepped inside and took a body bag from the cabinet, then followed them back into the house.

"I think it's going to be easier just to roll him up in a sheet," the deputy said. "The rigor mortis makes it tough to get 'em into one of those bags. The way his aim's bent, a sheet's just better."

"That's fine," I said. "Whatever's easiest." I just wanted it to be over.

We wrapped the sheet around him, then lifted him to the doorway and lowered him to the gurney. In the crowd, a baby cried.

"Where you take him?" a young woman called to us.

"To Culpeper," I answered. "To the hospital there."

"Hospital ain't gonna do him no good now," someone said, and there was a ripple of laughter that eased off into an uncomfortable silence.

I wanted to say something to them, to the women holding the babies, the dark-eyed children and the sullen, angry men. I stood for a moment, facing them. "I'm sorry," I said, finally, but they were already turning away.

We loaded him on the ambulance and marked en route to Culpeper Memorial Hospital. Joe and Norm rode up front.

"You want me to come back there with you?" Joe asked.

"No, I'm okay," I said.

"Well, I think I will anyway, if you don't mind."

"I don't mind," I admitted.

It was a quiet trip, interrupted only by sharp claps of thunder from a quickly passing storm. We traveled with the traffic, non-emergency, no lights or sirens.

I thought of my friend Bob Luckett, who worked as a paramedic for the city of Alexandria. "It's not the dead ones we pick up that get to me," he'd said. "It's not the ones we take away, it's the ones we have to leave behind."

Back then I could only listen to his experiences.

Now, I could understand.

"1050 just below the little lake on Route 3," the dispatcher announced. It was dusk on an August evening. Joe was still at his hardware store less than a mile from the accident site, so he responded to the scene.

"Overturned vehicle," he reported over his two-way. "Will advise on injuries."

Holly marked us en route, "Medic 291 responding."

"Persons trapped," Joe said. "Did you copy, 291?"

"291 copies," Holly said.

We were on the scene in less than a minute. The overturned vehicle was a convertible. I got off the ambulance while Holly and Purvis got the collars and backboards. I approached Joe, who was kneeling on the ground.

"Can you get to them?" I asked.

"I can't reach them but I can talk to them," he said. "They're both conscious."

I lay down on my stomach to try to get a look. "Is the car secure?" I asked Joe.

"It's wedged in the ground, Pat," he said. "It can't budge."

I eased myself partially under the car and looked down into the ditch. I could see the two men. Both were looking up at me. "My name is Pat," I said. "I'm with the rescue squad and we'll have you out of there real soon."

"That will be nice," the one closer to me said. His head was resting on a large cooler. The second man was further away from me. "Can you tell me your names?" I asked them.

"I'm Ron," the closer one said. "This is Eddie."

"Try not to move," I told them. "Where do you hurt?"

"My head," Ron told me, and I could see the blood on his forehead, matting his hair. "I think that's all."

"Eddie, what about you?" I asked.

"My arm feels broken, the one I'm lying on."

"Okay, just lie still," I said. "We'll get you out."

I backed away from the car and stood up. Joe was on the other side. "I think we can get them out over here," he called to me. "And Mac's here with the second ambulance."

We placed the backboard down on the ground and gently worked Eddie out and onto it. "Ah, fresh air," he said.

"Feels pretty good, doesn't it?" Sally said to him.

We collared him and moved him into the ambulance for a thorough secondary assessment, and Mac and Sally marked en route to Mary Washington Hospital. Ron was next. Getting him out was a little more difficult, because he was further away. We moved him out feet first, sliding him carefully onto the backboard. I could see that his hands were covered with blood.

"Is the blood on your hands from your head?" I asked him after we'd loaded him onto the ambulance.

"I think so," he said.

The laceration was about three inches long and right at the top of his head. I leaned forward to bandage the cut just as he reached up to feel the injury. "No, Ron," I said. "Move your hand so we can bandage it." His fingers brushed lightly over the wound, and that was all it took. The laceration was so deep that an artery had been nicked, but it had remained intact until Ron put his finger on it.

Blood began to gush out. I quickly covered it and applied direct pressure. "Purvis," I said, "let's move." We applied more bandages and maintained the pressure.

"What happened?" he asked us.

"Well, that cut you have just started to bleed a little more," Holly told him. I set up a line of Ringers, and then took a quick pulse. It was up to 110. I started the IV and then relieved Holly while she finished taking vitals. He was doing well, and the secondary assessment revealed nothing but some bruises and scraped knees.

"I can't believe how lucky they were," Holly said to us on our way home from the hospital. "To flip over in a convertible and land upside down on the one spot where there was room, and soft grass. What if they had landed in the road," she said.

"And what if the artery had severed the moment they wrecked," Purvis added.

"I don't even want to think about it," I said.

"What luck," Purvis said, nodding. "What unbelievable luck."

Their luck was good.

Hers was not.

It was three o'clock in the morning when the tones went off. "Overturned vehicle. Route 20. Lake of the Woods, your medic unit is due."

I knew that Jack was covering for Darren and Joe was on for Phyllis. But there was no CT around. I got out of bed and pulled on my jumpsuit. I was at the building within three minutes. Joe was already there, and Jack pulled in behind me. We heard the Mine Run fire engine announce they were en route to the scene.

I rested my head against the soft interior padding of the ambulance and closed my eyes. "I hope it's not bad," I said. "I'm tired and it's so cold outside."

It is so different running calls at night. I don't like it. The siren explodes around me, the sound amplified by the darkness. The lights turn the countryside crimson.

"Mine Run Engine 21 to Medic 29." I hear Brook's voice. "We got a possible 10-100 here," he said, "What's your location?"

Possible 10-100, possibly dead.

"Less than a mile away," Jack told him.

The overturned car was perched on an incline just beyond the shoulder of the highway.

Brook met me at the door of the ambulance. "She was thrown out, Pat," he said. "We can't find a pulse."

I couldn't see anything from the street.

"Pat," Brook said, as we approached the car, "she's pinned."

I stopped, confused. "I thought you said she was thrown out?"

He nodded. "She was thrown out."

"And she's pinned?"

"She's pinned underneath."

We walked around to the other side of the car. Lights from the engine illuminated the area. Her body rested on the incline. She was on her back, arms open, legs extended. She was very slender, very young. She still had shoes on, I remember, high heels. All of her was clear of the car except for her head.

I glanced at Brook, then approached the victim. I knelt down and felt for a radial pulse, because her arms were accessible. Nothing. I moved my hand slowly up to her shoulder, then to her neck. It was a tight squeeze between her neck and the roof of the car, but I could wedge my hand in there to check for a carotid. But, of course, there was nothing.

I stood up and moved away from the car.

Orange County deputy Dan Dixon was there. "Did you get anything?" he asked.

I shook my head.

"I didn't think so," he said. "Can you all take her to Clyde's after I get some pictures?"

Joe was beside me. "Just get a backboard and straps," I told him. "And some sheets. No sense bringing the gurney down here."

"We can't do anything until they get the car off of her," he said.

I guess I could have gone up to the ambulance. I could have waited there for them to bring the body to us. There was, after all, nothing to do but take her to Johnson's Funeral Home.

I didn't have to stay while Brook and Milt and the other firemen inflated the air bags and raised the car off her head. But I did.

And I didn't have to look at her.

But I did.

I thought of it later, lying in bed, unable to sleep.

It was not as I expected it would be. Across her forehead, on the left side, there was an indentation, deep and wide. That was all. There was no open injury on her face or the front of her head. In the back, her skull was cracked open, but we didn't see that until we turned her over onto the sheet.

Like strobes freezing motion, the salvos of light exploded from Dan's camera. But the motion was already frozen, never again to melt or thaw or stir.

It is an interesting thing, what can awaken a memory.

For Kirk, the smell of ashes and chimney residue.

For me, a crease, a furrow across my cheek from a wrinkled pillow-case I've slept on. It will be gone, erased before I finish my first cup of coffee. But my early morning reflection in the mirror takes me back, always.

Thirteen

During my Emergency Medical Technician course in 1981, the instructor warned us over and over about the differences between the classroom lessons and the real thing.

I'm not so sure any of us ever believed him. I know I didn't until a fellow named Shorty was thrown off his horse at a Texas rodeo. I had been an EMT for two days, and I was the only medically trained person there. When I stepped down from the bleachers to lend a hand, I thought that I would have at my disposal all the equipment necessary to care for an open fracture.

But there were no sterile four-by-fours, no padded board splints or triangular bandages. I fashioned splints from fence wood and a sling from someone's shirt and bandages from sweaty bandannas.

Now, when I tell my students "It's a whole different world out there," I don't think they believe me either.

Like most things, we all have to learn it on our own.

Madison County physician Jay Moscoe, like Dr. Schenck, is a country doctor. He's also an Advanced Cardiac Life Support instructor, and he worked with Mara and me on intubation techniques when we took the ACLS class.

Our airway manikin on the classroom table was at the perfect height for us to work and our intubation equipment was neatly aligned next to it.

"Select your blade and begin," he told me.

I finished the entire procedure in less than the fifteen seconds required.

"Good," he said. "Airway's secure."

Mara was next and she, too, finished with time to spare, graciously accepting his praise.

"Now, let's do it right," he told us.

"I thought we just did it right," I said.

He shook his head. "No, you did it correctly. Now, you'll do it right." He moved the manikin to the floor. "Bring all that stuff down here," he told us. "Then get down here on the floor."

We looked down at him.

"Come on," he insisted.

Mara and I knelt on the floor beside him. Then he lay down on his stomach. He patted the floor. "Right here."

The three of us lay stomach-down on the floor.

"This is the way it's going to be," he said. "Your patients aren't going to be lying on a table, are they?"

"No, I guess not," I told him.

"Of course not," he said. "Have you ever had a patient in cardiac arrest lying on a table?"

"No," I answered him, laughing.

"Mara," he said, facing her, "how about you?"

She shook her head and smiled at him. "Never."

"Okay," he said, turning back to me. "Pat, here you are lying on the bedroom floor. You're wedged between the bed and the woodstove and the dog is biting you in the butt. Now, intubate!"

He made his point.

Later, Mara and I realized we'd been lucky. There is a vomitus mix that comes with the airway manikin. We were at least spared that.

Taking his cue, I've added something to my EMT classes. Following their completion of CPR, we take Annie for a spin. We put her on a backboard and strap her to the gurney. They we go for a ride in the ambulance. One student performs CPR and one operates the bag mask. It's probably the part of the class they most remember. It certainly pinpoints the ones who will need Dramamine.

Twenty-two people started and finished the 1990-91 class. Of those, fourteen joined the rescue squad. Twelve became permanent members of a duty crew and five have already begun the Shock Trauma course.

Barbara was in that class, and Sally and Holly and Kirk. And Art, who plays drums in a bagpipe band. And Tom and Wes and Christie.

Our husband and wife team, Darren and Jerady, were there; and Kamryn, who captured Bobby's heart. And Donna.

"You're going to have to talk to Donna," Mara told me once. "She keeps giving her phone number out to our patients. Tell her she can't take everybody home with her."

"I'll tell her," I assured Mara.

And I did.

"The last patient I encouraged to call me," Donna explained, "was a young girl whose boyfriend keeps beating her. It was awful. She had bruises all over her."

"But Donna, unless you really know the people, sometimes it's not even safe."

"But it's so sad," she said to me, her eyes warm and empathetic.

"I know it is," I told her, "I often wonder myself where to draw the line."

"I'll be careful," she assured me. "I really will."

Donna is so good.

They all are.

"I was coming up the steps to class," Sally told me three weeks before the course ended, "and I could hear everybody talking and laughing and I just stopped on the landing . . . and listened . . . and realized how much everybody there meant to me and how much I was going to miss it."

"The class will end," I said to her, "but we'll all still be together."

She smiled. "For a long time, I hope."

I nodded. "I hope so, too."

It was early in January of 1991.

The call was for a forty-seven-year-old man who had fallen and possibly broken his ankle. A simple-sounding call. Christie was home from UVA, where she was working toward her masters in sports medicine.

"This is your call," I told her as we turned off of Route 20. "You can handle all the orthopedic injuries. You're the expert."

"Sounds good to me," she agreed.

"I'll take the call sheet in and you just tell us what to do."

"We're on the scene," Kirk called from the driver's seat.

"Want the oxygen to go in?" Joe asked her.

"Let's go in and see what we've got first," she answered him.

We stepped off the ambulance and approached the house. Just as we reached the door, a woman came toward us from the side yard. "You've got to help me," she pleaded. "I can't do anything with him."

"Where is he?" I asked.

"Inside," she said and she began to cry. "I have this bottle collection and he just started throwing them. Then he fell . . ."

"Does he have any weapons inside?" I asked, interrupting her.

"No," she cried. "Please help him. I told the dispatcher I think he broke his ankle when he fell. He's just sitting there on the floor."

"We will," I assured her. "We'll help him."

She opened the door to the kitchen. Before us, on the floor, sat her husband. He looked up at us through half closed eyes. I stepped over the pieces of glass and knelt down beside him. He smelled strongly of whiskey. "If you don't do something about this," he said, his words slurred, "this whole goddamned world is going to blow up."

"Do something about what?" I asked him.

He raised his cigarette to his lips and inhaled deeply.

"The war," he said, the smoke curling around his words.

I glanced at his wife.

"Henry," she said, "there isn't any war. The war's over."

I placed my hand on his. His pulse was strong. "Henry, did you hurt your ankle when you fell?" I asked him.

"I did." He nodded. "I hurt my ankle."

Christie knelt down and looked at his ankle. He grimaced when she touched it. I could see it was swollen. She asked Kirk to bring her a pillow and some cravats. "We're going to get it splinted for you," she said. "Then it will feel better."

"Okay," he said to her, despairingly.

"Henry, does anything else hurt you?" I asked.

"The war," was all he said. And he was crying.

We splinted his ankle and, because he had fallen, placed a collar on him and moved him onto a backboard before we lifted him to the gurney.

"He's got to get some help," his wife said to me as Joe and Kirk and Christie carried him to the ambulance. "He seems like he's coming apart."

"Do you have any idea why it's happening now?" I asked her.

"It's the Persian Gulf thing, Desert Shield," she said. "He stays glued to the TV all the time. He sits there drinking . . . and crying. Then, this morning, he just went crazy."

I put my arms around her. "I love him so much," she cried. "I just don't know what else to do."

"I'll see about getting him some help," I told her. "I'll tell the people in the emergency room."

"Thank you," she said. "I'll be there as soon as I can. I'm waiting on my neighbor to take me."

We pulled back onto Route 20 and headed toward Culpeper. He lay quietly on the backboard, tears running down his cheeks.

"Henry," I said to him, taking his hand, "is there anything that we can do to make you more comfortable?"

"It's going to be Armageddon all over again," he said. "I've told President Bush that. I write him letters all the time and you know what I get?"

"What?" I asked him.

He laughed. "I get a little card that says 'thank you for letting me know how you feel' or some shit like that. I get a thank you note. I can't believe it. I get a goddamned thank you note.

"He should have listened to me," Henry continued. "He wasn't in Vietnam. He didn't see what went on there. It's going to be another Vietnam," he said, crying again. "It's going to be another Vietnam."

His eyes reminded me of the eyes of my children long ago when they awakened in the darkness to nightmares, fiendish visions, and I would open my arms to them and hold them until the images were gone and they could sleep once more.

But I could do nothing to rid him of the horrors of his memories. And there was nothing I could say that would dispel his fear that the madness of the war in Vietnam was about to be repeated.

I talked to the emergency-room doctor about counseling for Henry.

"We'll see what we can do," he told me.

Two weeks later the United States launched massive air attacks against Iraq.

And I thought of Henry.

As it turned out, he had been wrong about Desert Storm becoming another Vietnam, but I wondered if that reality would be enough to drive away the demons.

He was already the casualty of one war.

I prayed he would not be the casualty of another.

It was the Monday before Thanksgiving and Kirk and I were cleaning the CPR manikins. He was unusually quiet, but I did not interfere with his silence. We are good friends and there is no urgency to fill all the empty spaces with talk.

I was putting the baby manikin back in the case when Kirk asked, "What was the worst call you ever had?"

I latched the case and set it down on the floor, thinking.

"I don't believe I can narrow it down to one," I said to him. "The house fire, of course, on Easter back in eighty-three." I sat down at the table. Kirk took the place across from me.

"That one stayed with me for a long time. The father was working in the garden and the mother had been taking clothes off the line when the propane heater exploded. The two small children were inside and there was no way she or her husband could get to them. The fire was so hot the firemen couldn't get close. We had to hold the mother to keep her from trying to get inside.

"We didn't have the stress debriefing then. We just had to work those things out for ourselves. But I was lucky," I told him. "I had people who'd listen to me."

"Even now with the debriefing, you've got to have people who will listen."

"That's right," I agreed.

Then I said to him, the memory still painful, "Jesse."

"The little boy in the wreck?"

"Yes. That was Jesse. That was the worst."

"When I was nine years old," he told me, "my father was killed in a hunting accident. It was the day after Thanksgiving. I was watching cartoons with my sister when we found out."

"Oh, Kirk," I said to him. "I'm so sorry."

"He died before he reached the hospital, maybe even before the rescue squad got him out of the field. And I sometimes wonder if the crew that was on that call, if someone years later asked them what their worst call was . . . if they'd say it was the one for my father.

"You've told us," he reminded me, "that what we are, the kind of people we are when we come into the rescue squad, that's who we'll be in the back of the ambulance."

I nodded remembering. "The goodness and the caring that is already there."

"Yes," he said, "and also our life's experiences. All the things that have helped to shape us, that affect our field of vision. Like my father. I am constantly reminded that the people we lose are not just flatline EKGs. They have families who loved them, families who must carry on with their lives, like my family did."

He met us at the front gate. "Hey," he greeted us. "I'm Herb Bateman. Mama's upstairs." Upstairs was four flights of narrow outside steps.

"We're going to need the chair stretcher," I said to Kirk.

Holly and I followed Mr. Bateman. "What exactly is wrong with her?" I asked him.

"She's just been sick," he responded. "The flu, I think. She's been vomiting a lot, hasn't eaten anything for three days."

"How old is she?"

"Eighty-three. It's just her and me now," he said, pausing on the third flight. "Daddy died five years ago and then my wife died last November. Don't have any kids. Just Mama and me."

We reached the house and walked in through the kitchen. He led us into the living room where we found her sitting in a rocking chair, quiet except for the sound of her breathing, shallow and labored. Her eyes were closed. I couldn't find a radial pulse, only a weak carotid.

Joe and Kirk came in with the chair stretcher. "Let's move her to the ambulance," I said. "I think that's going to be easier than trying to carry everything up here."

"I haven't been able to get her to eat a thing," her son said to me. "Even fixed her some rice pudding. She loves that. She likes it without the raisins. But she won't even eat any rice pudding."

Joe picked her up from the rocking chair and set her gently in the chair stretcher. She opened her eyes briefly and looked at him. Kirk put the straps around her and she patted his hand.

"Mr. Bateman, does she have any other medical problems?" I asked. "Heart disease, stroke, diabetes?"

"Her heart," he said, watching them carry her out of the living room. "She's had some problems with her heart. She takes fluid pills.

"I guess I'll just drive over," he said after he handed me the medicine. "I'm gonna shave and then I'll come straight on to the hospital."

"We'll see you there," I told him.

He smiled, "You tell Mama that, okay? Tell her I'll be right there."

I don't think he had any idea how serious her condition was.

Kirk and Joe and Holly were already in the ambulance when I opened the side door and stepped on.

"We've got problems," Kirk said. "She's completely unresponsive and we can only get a blood pressure of 80 palpation."

Joe filled the reservoir bag on the nonrebreather mask, then placed it on her face. "Her respirations are 36," he said.

"You ready?" Holly asked.

"Yeah," I said, and she backed the ambulance out of the driveway and turned toward Culpeper.

"Pulse is 124," Kirk said.

I started the IV and ran the fluids wide open, hoping to raise the blood pressure. Ten miles out of Culpeper, she stopped breathing. Then we lost her pulse. The EKG showed V-fib. I defibrillated three times and it went flatline.

"Start CPR," I said to Kirk while I reached for the Epi. Joe was ventilating.

They didn't work on her long in the emergency room.

"Her son thinks she just has the flu," Kirk said to me as we were changing the sheets on the gurney.

We wheeled the gurney out to the ambulance and looked toward the parking lot. He was there, walking toward us.

"Hey," he waved. "I brought Mama some rice pudding," he said, holding the dish up for us to see. "Should have brought some for everybody."

He stopped then, the smile fading from his lips. "What's wrong?" he asked us. "Has something happened to Mama?"

I couldn't say that someone else was taking care of her. None of us could.

"Mr. Bateman," I said, "I'm sorry."

He looked at each of us and his eyes filled with tears. "Mama's dead?"

I stepped forward and reached for his hand. "We'll go inside with you," I said to him.

We walked with him into the emergency room where we met the doctor.

Mr. Bateman turned away from us then, saying nothing, the plastic container of rice pudding still in his hand.

Fourteen

"I don't suppose you could cover for me tonight," Mara said. "I know it's short notice."

"I'd love to," I told her, "if you'll come over here and take charge of six fifteen-year-olds having a slumber party."

"Thanks anyway," she said. "Les and I will just wait until tomorrow night to go to the movie."

"Well, I hope you have a quiet night."

She laughed. "It'll probably be quieter than yours."

I hung up the phone and went into the living room to check on the girls. They'd finished the pizza and were stretched out on the floor, their attention focused on the television and the horror called Freddy.

"Ooooh," Jenny groaned.

"*Ooooh* is right," I said. "Why do you all watch that staff?"

"It's really neat, Mom," Jennifer said and the others moaned in agreement.

I shook my head in disbelief.

"Let me know if you need anything," I told them.

It was a warm night in the middle of Jane. I stuck my pager in the pocket of my shorts and stepped out on the back deck. A gentle wind stirred the leaves and the night sky glistened with stars. "I see the moon," I sang softly. It was not much more than a sliver, but it was enough to sing to. Nugget, our old golden retriever, rested his head in my lap.

The tones were a harsh sound against the peacefulness of the night. I pulled the pager from my pocket and listened.

"Attention Rescue 29 . . . you have a call on Flat Bottom Road . . . shooting."

"Oh, Mara," I said to the darkness. "So much for a quiet night."

They marked en route within three minutes, Mara and Tom and Judy and Donna. "Stand by at the church on the corner," the dispatcher told them, "until we're sure the scene is secure."

They were at the church for fifteen minutes before the deputy told them to come in.

"There was so much blood in his mouth," Judy told me later, "we thought it had been a suicide. We thought he'd shot himself in the mouth."

Tom was first to the car. He found the patient lying in the front seat. "It looked like he'd been sitting on the passenger side when he was shot and then had fallen across the seat."

"You want oxygen?" Donna asked.

"No," Mara said. "Let's just get him out of here."

"We were moving him out of the car," Judy said. "And this girl came out of the crowd. She walked over and looked down at him and said, 'Nope, nobody I know,' and then she just turned and walked away."

Donna told me, "It was so eerie. The car was lit up by lights from the police cars. We were in the middle of all that light and we couldn't see beyond it. Then Sheriff Spence told us that for our safety, he wanted us to hurry up and move him. They hadn't found the weapon and they didn't know who all was involved."

"We got him on the ambulance," Mara told me, "and then we took his clothes off. There was so much blood that at first we couldn't even find where he'd been shot.

"Finally, we saw it, in his chest. Then we figured that the blood and phlegm in his mouth and nose were from the lung trauma. It was awful."

"I got a weak carotid pulse when we first got on the scene," Tom said. "So we started CPR once we got him in the unit."

"We worked the code all the way to the hospital," Mara said. "I could never get an ET tube in. We just bagged him without it.

"He was only seventeen."

Mara would call me later that night. I would see Tom and Judy and Donna the next day. But then, sitting on the back deck of my house, all I knew was what I could hear from my pager . . . scene is secure . . . Medic 292 on the scene . . . Medic 292 en route to Culpeper working a full arrest . . .

I walked back in the house and into the kitchen for a cup of coffee. In the living room, the girls remained mesmerized by the movie they were watching, their blankets pulled up to their chins, tenuous protection against the grim madness.

I watched them while I listened to the voices coming sporadically from my pager, wishing there were some impenetrable blanket, some magic armor with which to cover them, to keep them forever shielded from the lunacy and the violence.

The Public Information Department of the Metropolitan District of Columbia Police reports that from January through November 1992, there were 332 gun-related homicides in Washington, D.C.

Sheriff Bill Spence tells me that during that same period of time, in Orange County, there was one. That one.

But even one is too many.

The call was for "a laceration."

Kathryn said, "Must be a bad one."

"Is the bleeding under control?" I asked the dispatcher.

"The caller didn't say," he responded.

"Rachel," I said, "get the trauma box out."

"I've got it ready to go," she answered.

"We're on the scene," Bobby announced.

We pulled into the driveway. Kirk was there just ahead of us. He was going up the steps with his first-aid bag in his hand. We followed him into the house.

I looked for spots of blood on the cream-colored carpet, but didn't see any. The patient was sitting on the sofa resting her head against her husband's shoulder, her legs elevated on the coffee table, her eyes closed. Kirk was examining her hand.

Rachel set the trauma box down on the floor and opened it.

I walked closer and looked. The laceration was on the tip of her left index finger.

"How did it happen?" I asked her.

"She cut it with a knife," her husband answered, "while she was peeling an apple."

"Was it bleeding badly?" Kirk asked.

She opened her eyes and answered him. "Yes, very badly."

"Is that why you put the rubber band around it?" I asked her.

She nodded.

"Well, I think we need to take it off," I said.

She pulled her hand away from Kirk. "No," she objected, "it will start to bleed again."

"She doesn't like to see the blood, you know," her husband said.

"I understand," I said. "But the end of her finger is purple, and cool, which means there is no circulation going there."

She looked at her husband. "What do you think?" she asked him.

He looked back at us. "The book said to use a tourniquet to stop the bleeding. Now you're telling us to take it off? I don't understand."

"Well, you're really just supposed to use a tourniquet as a very last resort," I said, "and never below the elbow or below the knee because you can do more damage than good."

"What if it starts to bleed again?" she asked, holding her hand against her chest.

"We'll bandage it," Rachel told her.

"Well," she finally consented, "all right."

Kirk gently unwrapped the rubber band from her finger.

"There," he said.

She looked down at her finger. A trace of blood oozed from the cut.

"See," she said, holding her finger up, as if to chastise us. "Look what you've done."

Rachel stepped forward with a Band-Aid.

"What if it comes off?" she asked as Rachel wrapped it snugly around her finger.

"We'll leave some extra ones here for you," I said.

I asked her if she would like for us to take her to the hospital, because we have to ask that of every patient.

And for a moment I thought she was going to say yes.

But her husband assured her he would care for her until the cut healed.

She signed the refusal, with her good hand, and Rachel gave her eight Band-Aids from the trauma box.

"It takes all kinds," Bobby remarked, pulling out of the driveway.

"Well, better now at two o'clock in the afternoon," Kathryn said, "than at two o'clock in the morning."

It was less than two weeks later when we got a second call to that residence. Her finger had healed, but she was vomiting and had a fever of a hundred and two.

"It's probably the flu," she said.

It was.

We lifted her onto the gurney and covered her with blankets. When we marked en route to Mary Washington Hospital, I glanced at my watch. It was 2:30 A.M.

Andy is one of our newest members. He is the younger son of my friends, Margaret and Mike Powers. He's a comic, and along with his sense of humor comes the ability to poke fun at himself which is an important prerequisite for survival.

He calls himself Mr. Response, and that he is.

"Can I go on this call?" he'll ask, popping up from nowhere.

All of us, if asked, would have to admit that we were once electrified by the flashing red lights and intoxicated by the piercing wail of the siren. It is not a fact that any one of us would be anxious to admit, but the thrill was there.

Andy is not hesitant at all. He is refreshingly honest about his enthusiasm. "Here I am," he announces. "Mr. Response is ready to go."

Now, he is a driver. CPR is his only medical skill. The day after he finished his course, he was the second one on the scene of a call for cardiac arrest. Art did ventilations. Andy did compressions.

Soon he will be in my EMT class. I will get to watch him grow and mature, and that is as exciting to me as the lights and sirens are to him.

"Andy's a lot like I was," Bobby said to me, "when I first joined."

I smiled at him. "In what way?" I asked, already knowing.

"He's so . . . excited."

"Um-hum." I nodded. "He is very much like you were. You drove us all a little crazy," I said to him. "You had a million questions and lots of big ideas."

He chuckled. "Yeah."

"But," I continued, "you started to grow on us just like Andy has. And we realized that some of your ideas were good ones.

"You just needed a little of the newness to rub off."

I am no longer new.

I am one of three life members who are still active on the squad. That's ten years. Plus.

I can't remember when I first became aware that my "newness" was fading. I can't put an hour or a date on the moment when the luster began to fade, when I realized that the siren had become, at times, more an irritant than a stimulant.

Dr. Schenck tells us that the journey of a volunteer rescue squad member begins with frenzied enthusiasm and ends, after some period of time, with a struggle just to survive.

"Maybe that's why we have our Andys," I suggested to him. "As a reminder."

"Maybe so," he agreed.

So I try not to be too judgmental with Andy. I try not to force sensitivity upon him. I praise him for his driving skills and I encourage him in his studies. And each time he pops up from nowhere, uniform in hand, eyes sparkling with frenzied enthusiasm, shouting, "Can I go on this call?" I am reminded.

I tell my new EMTs, "Try to stay calm."

Bob Luckett used to say, "Don't get the big eye."

And Dr. Schenck reminds us, "It's not your emergency. It's theirs."

It was a lazy July afternoon, and Jennifer and I were trying to coax Nugget outside for a bath. As soon as he sees the hose, he flattens to the ground, and we have to carry him the rest of the way. We were at that point in the process when the phone rang.

"Just let it ring," I told Jennifer, my arms around Nugget. We were less than ten feet away.

"Oh, Mom," she objected, "it might be Jenny. She was going to call me from her grandmother's house."

"Okay," I conceded. "Just hurry up."

She ran toward the house and disappeared inside. But within moments, she was back.

"It's for you," she said.

"Can you tell them to call back?" I asked. "We're kind of busy here."

"Mom, whoever it is really sounds upset."

I looked down at Nugget. "You put someone up to this, didn't you, you cowardly dog." I let him go, and he quickly bolted away.

Jennifer shook her head. "Now we're going to have to start all over," she complained.

"Hey," I said, "who had to answer the phone?"

I walked into the kitchen and picked up the receiver.

"Hello."

"Pat?"

"Yes, this is Pat."

"You've got to come help me," the man said. "I need a CT."

At first I thought it was a joke. I didn't recognize the voice and it sounded a little like he was laughing.

"Who is this?" I asked. Jennifer looked at me and I winked at her. "Sounds like somebody's playing a joke," I whispered.

"Pat," the man said again. "It's Norm."

"Norm?"

"Yes, I've been stung by a bee, Pat. You've got to come help me."

"Norm!"

Then I realized he hadn't been laughing. He was wheezing so badly it sounded like laughter.

"Where's Jackie?" I asked.

"She's on her . . . way home. She'll be . . . here in just . . . a minute." He could barely get his breath.

"You haven't called the squad?" I asked him. I'd had my pager with me and I hadn't heard the tones.

"No," he said. "I called . . . you."

"Norm, don't you have your EpiPen?"

"It's . . . expired."

"Okay, Norm, sit down. I'll call for the ambulance. I'm on my way."

I called.

The dispatcher answered, "Fire and Rescue."

"I need an ambulance," I blurted out.

"Where?"

114

My mouth was so dry.

"At Norm Ensrud's house."

"Where?"

"Norm Ensrud!"

"Spell the name please."

"E-N-S-R-U-D."

"That's E-S-R . . ."

"No, Ensrud, Ensrud, E-N-S-R-U-D. He's been stung by a bee."

"He's what?"

"STUNG BY A BEE!"

"Okay. The address?"

Oh, what was his address? "Jennifer," I shouted, "hand me the directory."

"What, Mom?" she called back to me.

"THE DIRECTORY!"

"Where is it?"

"Ma'am, I need the address."

"Just a minute," I told him, then put my hand over the receiver and yelled to Jennifer. "It's on my desk."

Skyline. That's it. Skyline.

"SKYLINE!" I blurted into the phone.

"Numericals?"

"I don't know . . . just tone them out . . . I'll know it when I see it."

"Ma'am, I'll need the numericals."

"JUST TONE THEM OUT!"

I met the ambulance at the building and climbed in the back. "Let's go," I said.

"Where?" Joe asked.

"To Norm's," I shouted.

Joe looked puzzled. "It's at Norm's? The dispatcher said 'Esrue.'"

"Trust me," I told him. "It's at Norm's."

"Is he okay?" Purvis asked.

"He's allergic to bees," I said. "He's not okay."

He was covered with hives when we got there. Jackie had put a cold cloth on his head and he was stretched out on the sofa. His respirations were 42 and very labored.

I knelt beside him. "Norm," I asked, "where were you stung?"

"In the mouth," he said. He was barely able to move his lips, they were so swollen. His eyes were red and puffy, little more than slits. "It was in my can of Pepsi."

I quickly called the hospital and got orders for Epi and Benadryl.

"He's not wheezing as badly," Joe said to me as I was drawing up the Epi in the syringe.

"Could be because his airway is closing," I snapped.

I injected the Epi and picked up the second syringe with Benadryl and injected that.

"My CT," Norm whispered, breathing easier.

"Oh, yes," I agreed, giving him a hug.

"Another save," Joe said, smiling.

And Jackie gave him a great big kiss. "You don't have to tell me to pucker up," Norm said, laughing. "I'm already puckered."

So I tell my classes, "Stay calm."

I tell them what Bob said. "Try not to get the big eye. It's not your emergency. It's theirs."

I even add, "Before you take your patient's pulse, take your own."

I apologized to my crew.

"You were a terror," Joe said.

"I know," I admitted. "It was so difficult hearing Norm like that. It's so hard when it's one of ours."

"Yes, it is," he nodded.

"I'll be better next time," I told them.

"I hope there won't be a next time," he said.

"Well, I made Norm promise to get a new EpiPen. So if we can keep everybody else safe and healthy, we'll be fine."

"How nice that would be if we could."

"Yes," I agreed. "It would be wonderful."

But it wasn't to be.

Fifteen

In Austintown, Ohio, in the summer of 1990, thirty-nine-year-old Kathy Price was diagnosed with immune deficiency chronic pneumonia.

"It's your breast implants," she was told, "and will most likely also impair your central nervous system." The silicone toxicity ultimately produced stroke-like symptoms, transient episodes of paralysis, and blank spaces in her mind.

"Your life expectancy," her doctor said, "is six months."

"I want us to go ahead with our trip," she told her husband that night.

"I don't know, Kathy," he said.

"I'll be fine," she persisted. "It's all planned for September. That's less than two months away."

So, against her doctor's advice, seven weeks later they flew to Mexico's Yucatán Peninsula. On the plane, Kathy read an article in a travel magazine about a gift shop on an island near Cancún. She showed her husband the article. "Bob," she asked, "can we go?"

"If you feel up to it," he nodded. "Of course."

The next day they drove from Cancún to Punta Sam, where they caught the ferry that traveled the eight miles to the island of Isla Mujeres. When he tried to persuade her to sit in the car for the forty-five minute trip across the bay, she refused. "There's too much to see," she said. She took his hand and they walked up the narrow iron steps to the upper level of the ferry, and she breathed in the sweet sea air.

Only five miles long, Isla Mujeres is set like a gem in the turquoise waters of the Caribbean. The gift shop, La Loma, is on the Main Square. The shop's owner, Judith Fernandez, welcomed them warmly. *"Hola,"* she nodded, smiling.

"¡Hola!" Kathy responded, then shrugged her shoulders. *"No comprende español,"* she said apologetically.

"It's all right," Judith laughed. "I understand English. Please, make yourselves at home. Look around."

They did, admiring the rich tapestry of the blankets, the intricate patterns of the paintings and jewelry, and the masks, illustrating the continuing Mayan influence. They browsed for forty-five minutes, then spent another two hours just talking with Judith about the Mayan Indians. She encouraged them to visit the ruins of Chichén Itzá and the Mayan Temple Ixchel.

"There are practically no Mayan names left," Judith told them. "The Spanish renamed the towns as they conquered them."

"Isla Mujeres means the Island of Women," she explained. "In 1517, Francisco Hernandez de Cordova sailed from Cuba in search of slaves and land. When he reached this island in the Yucatán Peninsula, he found idols of goddesses of the country. In fact, he found so many statues of women," she said, "that he named our island the Island of Women, Isla Mujeres."

When the two women parted that day there was a great sadness. Kathy, conscious of her own destiny, feared she would never see Judith again. Her eyes remained fixed on the island as the ferry carried them away.

Perhaps, when one is aware of the brevity of one's days, one has a renewed sense of being and of purpose.

The next day, she told Bob, "I have to go back."

When Kathy arrived back at La Loma, Judith greeted her at the door as if she'd been expecting her. "We have much to do," Judith said. They talked most of the day about the island and the needs of the people there. "Books for the children," Judith said. "A school so they can have a future." In peaks of excitement and enthusiasm, Judith would slip back into her native language, and the women would laugh together, wonderful, rich laughter that accompanies happy moments of shared friendship.

"I will see you soon," Kathy told Judith when they said good-bye that day. Kathy was determined to face this misfortune in her life with the courage with which she'd faced the breast cancer, and, when she left the island, she knew she had to prove the doctors wrong.

"Judith is right," Kathy said to Bob. "There is much to do."

For the next ten months, she collected materials for the school, books and educational toys, paper and pencils and crayons. Twice, she traveled back to the island, the second time for a tour of the school that she had helped to create.

Kathy was in pain most of the time, and had been hospitalized three times with pneumonia, but she was determined to return in mid-July with additional boxes of supplies.

On July fourth, all across the United States, Americans were celebrating Independence Day. It had been twenty-six days since the Rescue Museum had opened in Roanoke, Virginia, and Dave Murray was spending a quiet holiday with his wife and children. Conover Hunt was making final travel plans for a much-needed vacation.

In Austintown, Kathy Price sorted through school books and used clothes.

I was on rescue duty. We only had one call, for a ten-year-old who'd cut his hand on a broken pickle jar.

On that same day, on the island of Isla Mujeres, Judith Fernandez was cleaning out her bedroom closet. She stood on a wooden chair she'd pulled in from the dining room, reached for a shoebox on the top shelf, and lost her balance, falling hard on the tile floor and shattering her hip.

Because of that moment, all our futures would be redefined.

The call was for "chest pains."

The dispatcher gave us directions.

"It's quite a distance," I told Dick. "It's probably going to take us twenty minutes to get there."

I switched on the siren at the intersection and we headed south on Route 20.

"Do you have any more patient information?" I asked the dispatcher.

"All we have," she said, "is a sixty-eight-year-old male with chest pains."

"Any cardiac history?" I asked.

"Caller wasn't sure."

Several cars ahead of us pulled over so we could pass.

"I don't like this," Joe said from the back of the ambulance.

"Being so far away?"

"Yeah."

"Neither do I," I told him. "If he's having a heart attack, a lot can happen before we get there."

It was twenty-two minutes before we arrived on the scene. Joe and I got off the ambulance with the lifepack and oxygen, then Dick backed the ambulance into the driveway.

"Rescue squad," I announced, knocking on the screen door.

"Door's open," a woman shouted from inside.

We walked into the small living room and saw our patient lying on the sofa. The woman sat in a chair across the room, her heavy arms folded across her chest.

"Good morning," I said, approaching the man. "How do you feel?"

"Not so good," he answered, rubbing his hand across his chest. "I've got this pain."

Joe knelt beside him. "I'm going to give you a little oxygen."

"Well, thank you," the man said.

I put my hand on his and felt for his pulse. It was regular and 76. His skin was dry and he was breathing easily. Joe placed the nasal cannula on him.

"Y'all sure don't have much to do with your time," said the woman.

"Ma'am?" I asked, turning toward her.

"You heard me," she said, cocking her head to one side.

I nodded. "Yes, ma'am, I heard you. I wasn't sure if you were talking to us."

"She's talking to you all right," the man said. "She just doesn't think I'm sick."

I glanced at Joe, then turned back to our patient.

"Have you ever had a heart attack?" I asked him.

He shook his head. "Nope."

"Do you have any heart problems?"

"Shit, no," the woman muttered.

"I don't know," he said, ignoring her. I followed his lead and ignored her, too.

"Describe the pain for me," I asked.

He shrugged his shoulders. "It hurts," he said. "Is that what you mean?"

"No," I told him. "I mean, is it dull or sharp. Does it feel like pressure on your chest, and is the pain anywhere other than your chest?"

"It's in his head," me woman grumbled.

Joe rested his hand on my shoulder. "Dick and I will bring in the gurney," he said.

I nodded.

We were all getting pretty good at ignoring her.

"Sharp," the man exclaimed. "That's it. Like a stitch in my side. Only it's in my chest. Just like before."

"Before?"

"Yeah," he said.

"How often do you have these pains?" I asked him.

"Right often."

"What do you do to make it better?" I asked. "Do you take medicine to make me pain go away?"

"Ginger ale and beer," me woman answered.

I thought I had misunderstood. "Ginger ale and beer?" I asked.

He grinned at me. "You gotta go with what works," he said.

"We're having some trouble getting the gurney inside," Joe said to me through me screen door.

"He can walk," was the woman's suggestion.

I was inclined to agree with her.

"Did you try the ginger ale and beer this morning when your chest started to hurt?" I asked.

He glanced quickly at the woman and then looked back at me. "Couldn't," he said.

"Why not?"

"I'm out of beer."

"Pat," Joe said, "do you want the chair stretcher?"

"He can walk," the woman barked.

"I can walk," the man agreed, standing up.

"If walking makes it worse," I told him, "sit down and we'll . . ."

"Ahh," the woman growled, "quit babying him."

"I'm fine," he said. "I'm feeling good now."

"Go to work then," she said.

"Well, now," he said, walking toward the door. "I might as well go to the hospital now that the ambulance is here."

"Suit yourself," she yelled as the screen door slammed shut behind him.

"Ain't she something," he said to us as we traveled toward Culpeper. "Ain't she a prize. Lord, I do love her so."

"Some things are just not worth trying to understand," I said as we headed down Route 3 on our way back home. "Just not worth it."

"The whole thing gave me a headache," said Dick.

"I don't know how you kept a straight face," Joe said to me. "If I hadn't gone out for the gurney, I probably would have fallen on the floor laughing."

"No, you wouldn't," I told him. "You would never do that, no matter how absurd it got."

"You're sure of that?"

"Well, almost."

But I am sure.

We save our laughter for later.

Just as we save our tears.

It was a warm Sunday morning, a lazy kind of day. I carried my coffee out on the deck. Blooms on the dogwood and redbud trees sparkled in the bright rays of the morning son. Song sparrows pulled sunflower seeds from the feeder by my kitchen window. I waved to my neighbor across the street and sipped my coffee.

The tones caught me off guard.

I ran inside, dropped my cup in the sink, and grabbed my uniform. The dispatcher announced that the call was "at the Burbank residence."

"At the Burbank residence." Phyllis has been stung by a bee, I thought to myself. She's planting flowers . . . it's happened before. She's allergic to bee stings, but that's easy to fix. Epi, Benadryl. Easy to fix . . . easy to fix . . .

". . . for a possible heart attack," the dispatcher continued.

"It can't be," I whispered to myself as I hurried toward the station.

I pulled into the parking lot. Kirk was already there. And Joe. Sally pulled in behind me. Then Jim. I climbed up front and reached for the radio.

"Everybody on?" I asked.

"Yeah," Joe yelled from the back. "Let's go."

Kirk accelerated out of the driveway and we headed down Lakeview Parkway.

"Medic 293 is en route," I told the dispatcher.

He replied, "Medic 293. Just received a call from one of your members on the scene . . . it's Mr. Burbank . . . CPR is in progress."

"No," Jim said.

I blinked back the tears that burned my eyes.

"Medic 293, were you direct?"

"Yes," I acknowledged, my voice, my heart breaking.

Phyllis was in my EMT class. She joined the squad eight months after I did. We became cardiac technicians together. For a long time, she was our squad's only CPR instructor. She is as creative as anyone I've ever known. She paints and works with ceramics and creates wonders outside with plants and flowers. She is inquisitive and funny and she is so very, very kind.

She was sitting on the arm of the sofa when we rushed into their house. I wished for time to stop, to hold her, but there wasn't any time. She pointed down the hall toward their bedroom. "Dick's in there," she told us.

It all seemed unreal in that room, so cramped and hot. Bobby and Dan were doing CPR. The monitor showed ventricular fibrillation. I pressed the paddles against his chest and fired once, then again, and again.

Bill arrived. Then Barbara and Christie, who went to Phyllis. I started the IV and gave Epi, and Bill defibrillated. Then lidocaine and defibrillation again.

"Let's move him out," I said.

They lifted him onto a backboard, continuing CPR, and started down the hallway. I walked ahead of them back to the living room, where Barbara was sitting with Phyllis.

I sat down next to them on the sofa. "What happened, Phyllis?" I asked her, looking for some clue.

"We went to West Virginia yesterday to look at our property there. He seemed a little quiet," she said, "but he didn't let me know anything was bothering him until we got up this morning. He'd never had any problems with his heart. Then the pain got so bad, he just fell over."

"Oh, Phyllis," I said, taking her hand.

"I'll drive you to the hospital," Barbara told her.

"No," she said, slowly shaking her head. "Thank you, but I think I'd like to go on the ambulance. Pat, is that all right?"

"Whatever you want to do is all right," I said. "I just don't want it to be too difficult for you."

"I started CPR on him," she said softly. "Nothing could be much more difficult than that."

Barbara walked her to the ambulance, helped her into the front, and tightened the seat belt on her.

I got in the back with Dick.

Seven months before this April day, he had retired as battalion chief after serving twenty-five years with Fairfax County Fire and Rescue. He had once been chief of our Fire Department. He was only fifty-three years old. He and Phyllis had tickets for a November Caribbean cruise. They were planning to build a house on their land in West Virginia.

We worked on him all the way to Mary Washington Hospital with Phyllis just an arm's length away. Halfway there, we lost all rhythm on the monitor.

Phyllis never asked us any questions.

"I knew," she said later, "from the very beginning."

I suppose we all did.

Uniformed fire and rescue personnel from Lake of the Woods and from Fairfax County crowded into the chapel at Johnson's Funeral Home for Dick's funeral.

Rev. Glen Cannon spoke. "The Bible tells us," he said, "that we won't know the day or the hour when death will come." He looked around the room, an easy, gentle smile crossing his face. "This, of course, is no news to the people in this room. All of you know," he said, "that when the call comes, when the tones go off, you go.

"The problem is," he continued, "sooner or later you have to face the fact that there's a call that just doesn't work, a person you just can't save. And it is very important that you know and that you always remember . . . it doesn't mean you've failed."

All around that small wooden chapel, faces were upturned. Ears were hungry for the words they were hearing. And hearts, yearning for peace, began to heal.

Sixteen

"DAVE MURRAY," I exclaimed, pleased to hear his voice. I hadn't talked with him since the opening of the Rescue Museum. "How've you been?"

"Busy," he said. "I've got a lot to tell you."

And he did. He talked to me for almost an hour about two women named Kathy Price and Judith Fernandez.

It was an incredible story.

Judith lay still on the floor. Marguerita, the girl who came in to help her twice a week, found her there.

"Ambulancia," Judith pleaded. *"Por favor."*

The phone lines did not go far enough from Judith's house to reach the Red Cross, so Marguerita had to call the taxi company and pray that someone was there to answer.

"Call the Red Cross and ask them to send an ambulance," Marguerita told the man who answered the phone.

Judith was in excruciating pain. Even the slightest movement was unbearable.

"The ambulance boys finally came," Judith said later. "The old truck they had broke down twice on the way to my house. And they didn't have the proper supplies. They were almost as scared as I was."

Without adequately supporting her leg, they lifted her from the floor to the gurney. "I almost passed out with the pain," she recalled.

Then they had to wait for the ferry.

When Kathy called several days later to let Judith know when she would be arriving with the supplies, she had no idea what had happened to her friend. It took almost an hour to get all the information and to track down Judith in the hospital in Cancún.

"I'll be able to leave in ten days," Judith told Kathy, "but I still won't be able to walk."

"Not to worry," Kathy said. "I'll be there."

Ten days later, when Judith was released, Kathy was there to meet her. In addition to the clothes and books and assorted school supplies, she also brought a wheelchair.

She took her friend home to Isla Mujeres.

Judith was mending, but her recovery was far from over. She would need another operation and more therapy. The scars on her leg would fade, but they would never disappear. Neither would her limp.

Kathy was troubled for her friend, and she was also quite mindful of the fact that at any moment, someone else on the island could be injured or become terribly ill, and, like Judith, would be without adequate prehospital care.

Dave paused in his telling of the story. "Now," he said, taking a deep breath, then exhaling slowly, "this is the part you're just not going to believe."

The week passed quickly on Isla Mujeres. Kathy was to board the plane for Miami the next morning, then travel back to Ohio. Judith was sleeping soundly, and Kathy wrote her a brief note, "Gone for a walk. Be back soon."

She walked through the narrow streets where there is always the musty smell of the sea. She wandered past the small and humble dwellings and greeted each passing islander, "*Hola.*"

They smiled broadly and returned her salutation, "*¡Hola!*"

Kathy approached the beach, slipped off her shoes, then stepped onto the sand. In the distance, across the blue Caribbean water, she could see the sharp outlines of the buildings in Cancún's hotel zone. Tiring, she stopped at the Cristalmar to rest.

She ordered a glass of pineapple juice and sat down at a table facing the ocean, propped her feet up in the chair next to her, and stared out at the azure sea.

"Isn't it breathtaking?" remarked the woman next to her.

Kathy, deep in thought, had not noticed her until she spoke.

"Yes," Kathy nodded. "I've never seen anything more beautiful."

"I haven't either," the woman said, smiling. "Not even in Texas. Are you vacationing?" she asked.

"No," Kathy answered. "I'm visiting a friend who had an accident."

"I'm sorry," she said. "I hope it wasn't anything serious."

Kathy, suddenly overcome with fatigue and sadness, began to cry.

The woman reached in her purse for a tissue and handed it to her. "Is there anything I can do?" she asked.

"No," Kathy said, drying her tears. "Not unless you have an ambulance."

"An ambulance?"

"Yes," Kathy nodded. "My friend fell and there was no decent ambulance," she explained. "It just doesn't seem fair . . . what we have at home in the United States doesn't even exist here."

"Well," the woman said, leaning closer, "I don't have an ambulance, but I might know someone who does."

"You're kidding?" Kathy laughed, "I must be dreaming."

The woman laughed too, then reached back into her purse and pulled out her wallet. She took a card and handed it to Kathy.

"Okay, Pat," Dave said, "you know whose name was on the card?"

"Whose?" I asked.

"Mine!" he said. "My name."

"Well, who was me woman?" I asked him. "And why did she have your card?"

He told me, "It was Conover Hunt."

On an island of 14,000 people and sixteen hotels, Kathy Price had sat down next to Conover Hunt.

"It was a miracle," Kathy told Dave the following week when she called him. "Nothing short of a miracle."

"I can get an ambulance," Dave told her, "for $7500. It's used, but the ad says it's in good shape."

"I don't have seventy-five cents to buy an ambulance," she told him, "much less $7500."

"Okay," he assured her. "I'll look around. I'll see what I can do."

"You're an angel," she told him.

He did it.

It took only a few phone calls before Dave learned that Catawba-Masons Cove Volunteer Rescue Squad had a 1978 ambulance they were going to sell. He immediately approached the chief, Don Jones.

"Pat," Dave said, "with a story like this, how could anyone say no?"

Don Jones couldn't.

On December 12, Dave called Kathy.

"*Feliz Navidad,*" he greeted her. "*Yo tango una ambulancia par ete.*"

"Dave," she said. "Is that you?"

"Kathy," he laughed. "You still haven't learned Spanish?"

"No," she told him. "I just haven't gotten around to it. What did you say?"

"I said 'Merry Christmas,' Kathy. Your ambulance is here."

On December 23, a cold and cloudy winter day, in front of the Rescue Museum in Roanoke, Virginia, Dave Murray held a press conference, and he and Don Jones presented Kathy Price with the keys to the ambulance.

"*Feliz Navidad,*" Dave said to her.

She hugged him tightly. "I know what that means now," she said. Then she faced the reporters, "It will be the merriest of Christmases for the people of Isla Mujeres," she said, "because of the kindness of Dave Murray and the Julian "Wise Foundation and the Catawba-Masons Cove Rescue Squad."

"So, Pat," he said, his story finished, "what do you think?"

"I think that if I hadn't believed in miracles before, I'd sure believe in them now," I told him. "That is really incredible."

"Isn't it?" he agreed. "And I really did feel like Santa Claus."

"I'm sure," I told him. "I feel like you've given me a gift just in telling me about it. You know, this is the greatest tribute you could pay to Julian Wise. It's everything he believed in."

"Yes," he said softly. "I think he'd really be pleased. But unfortunately, getting the ambulance to Mexico was the easy part. The red tape there was endless, and the ambulance is still tied up in customs near Cancún. It hasn't even made it to the island," Dave said," and I have no idea when they'll get it out. When we do, I'd like for you to help with the next stage."

"What is that?" I asked.

"We need some instructors to teach the people there how to use the equipment on the ambulance," he said.

"You mean — " I began.

"Yep," he interrupted me, "I want you to go to Mexico."

"Mexico?"

"Mexico!" I shouted, an affirmation for my mother and for me. "I still can't believe it."

My father picked up the extension. "Hi, sweetie," he greeted me.

I no longer began each conversation with him with a hurried "how are you?" He was good. I could hear it in his voice. All his checkups had been excellent, and his exercise routine was going well.

"Hi, Daddy," I said. *"Qué pasa?"*

"I thought I was supposed to ask you that," he said, laughing.

"I'd let you," I told him, "but that's all the Spanish I know."

"Well, tell us about this trip," he said.

"Not much to tell about right now," I responded. "About all I know is that I'm going."

"You better get some Spanish books from David," my mother suggested.

"Not a bad idea," I said.

The next night, I called David in Austin.

"He's teaching his GED class tonight," Andy told me.

David and Andy had graduated from James Madison University the year before and were working together in VISTA.

"You guys doing okay?" I asked him.

"Great," he said. "They're keeping us busy but we love it."

David wrote me long, newsy letters filled with descriptions of his work there and of the poor and neglected people.

"I need a quick course in Spanish," I told Andy and then I explained why.

"That's great," he responded. "You and David are both going south of the border. When do you leave?" he asked.

"I'm not sure," I said. "Lots of details to work out first. Be nice if David and I could start out together, wouldn't it?"

"It would be perfect," he agreed. "Did he tell you that he and Matt and I are thinking about traveling west this summer, out to Washington?"

"Matt mentioned it in his last letter," I said. "Jack Kerouac has really gotten to you all, hasn't he?"

Andy laughed. "How'd you guess?"

"I've read his book," I told him. "I think the trip sounds wonderful, Andy. So wonderful I'm envious," I admitted.

Before I hung up, I asked Andy to give David my love and tell him I'd call back soon.

In the winter of 1971, David was two and Matt just seven months. While their father was away on business, we visited my parents in Salem. On our second day there, David and my mother awoke early. She fixed his breakfast and sat at the table across from him while he ate. He took a sip of orange juice and then set the glass down hard on the table, splashing juice on the tablecloth.

"Nana," he said, looking toward her, "Help me."

She pushed back her chair and hurried to him. His eyelids fluttered, then closed. He fell into her arms.

I awoke to my mother's voice. "Something's wrong with David!"

I held him tightly in my arms as my father rushed us to the hospital.

"Please don't let him die," I cried, helpless, unable to do more.

Before we reached the downtown hospital, he opened his eyes.

"Mama," he said, touching my cheek with his small hand.

His BEG showed a slight irregularity, indicating he'd had a seizure. Perhaps a once-in-a-lifetime incident, the doctors told us. He seemed fine. And he was. We were home by noon.

It wasn't until years later that I realized that if he hadn't been fine, I wouldn't have known what to do.

"Something's wrong with David," my mother had said.

And all I could do was beg him not to die.

What if his breathing had stopped? Or his heart?

I knew no CPR.
I could not have saved my son.

David was eight weeks old when Apollo II landed on the moon, and I carried him out into our front yard in Chapel Hill, North Carolina. "Look up, David," I said softly, leaning back in my chair so his eyes faced heavenward. "There is a man walking on the moon," I told him. "Anything is possible, David. Anything."
And he heard me.

I cannot imagine a world without him, without his friendship, his humor, his songs, and his poetry, and his determination to make life better for those who have so little.
Just as I cannot imagine my life without Matt and Jennifer.

Barbara often runs calls with the squad in the town where she works. Last week, she ran a call there for an automobile accident. The woman in the car had some facial lacerations and a broken arm. Her twelve-year-old did not fare so well. He wasn't wearing a seat belt, and he was ejected from the car. Squad members did everything they could, but the boy was pronounced dead at the hospital.
She called me late that night. "I had an awful call today," she said. "Do you have time to hear about it?"
I'd heard the pain in her voice. "Of course I do," I said.
"I left the hospital before they told his mother," she said. "But some-one told me later that when they told her, you could hear her scream-ing all the way out in the parking lot.
"A seat belt would have saved him. A seat belt. I just can't imagine not having Shelly," she said. "I can't imagine losing my child; but to lose my child and then know I could have done something to prevent it, I couldn't live with that."

So we preach prevention. Learn CPR. Wear your seat belt. Have a designated driver. Don't smoke.
For a long time, I encouraged my parents to take a CPR course. I finally decided, if I couldn't get Mohammed to the mountain, I would bring the mountain to Mohammed. Christmas 1990, along with the kids and the dog and the presents, I wedged Annie into the car.

"Merry Christmas," I said, pulling Annie from her black case and stretching her out on the floor. "Welcome to CPR class."

There are no guarantees in life.
So we don't promise everyone will be saved.
But we do promise that everyone will have a better chance.
In fact, we guarantee it.

The living room was richly decorated with antiques and I was acutely aware of the mud on my shoes as I sat in the velvet-and-gold brocade chair. The deputy sat across from me on the sofa, taking information from our patient's wife.

We'd given him a choice, us or the police. He'd chosen the latter.

"I don't need a rescue squad," he'd argued. "I'm not hurt."

"You almost were," his wife said, her voice shaking.

She'd started looking for him after she spotted the note on the kitchen table.

"I'm a failure," it read. "I'm sorry. You'll be better off without me."

She found him in the garage in the driver's seat of the BMW, his hands tightly gripping the steering wheel. She reached across him and switched off the ignition, then quickly opened the garage door. The cold December rain splashed against her as she breathed in the frigid air, but she welcomed the cold and the rain and the wind, for it would drive the deadly carbon monoxide away from her husband.

"Times are hard," the man said, interrupting the deputy. He was in a chair that matched mine, gold and velvety. He hadn't said much. His wife had done most of the talking, and she and the deputy talked about him in the third person, as if he weren't there.

He'd made the decision to go with the deputy to the Mental Health Clinic in Orange, and I handed him our call sheet.

"This just says flat we offered to take you to the hospital and you refused," I explained, handling him the pen and showing him where to sign.

He smiled warmly at me. "I hope you're not mad," he said, and his voice sounded hollow. "I'm sure you all are very nice. I just have never cared very much for medical things." He signed the call sheet and handed it back to me.

"I'm not mad," I told him, gently touching his hand. "I just want you to be all right."

Outside, the cold rain continued. I ran from the porch to the ambulance where Joe and Kirk were waiting. Joe opened the side door for me and I stepped inside.

"The deputy's going to take him to the clinic now," I told them, shaking the rain from my hair.

Kirk glanced back at the house as we pulled away. "Looks like they have everything, doesn't it?"

"Looks can be deceiving," I said. "Remember Richard Cory?"

Joe shook his head. "A patient?" he asked.

"No," I said, smiling. "A poem. About a man who had everything; money, status, everything. And he shot himself."

We pulled back into the bay. I glanced at my watch. Forty-five minutes from start to finish. Forty-five minutes before, I didn't know this man, had not seen his elegant house, would not have recognized his BMW. But he'd stepped into my life and etched his suffering into my memory.

Almost twelve years.

How many lives by now, I wonder. Fifteen hundred? Two thousand? More?

Lives intertwined with mine.

Strangers . . . whose pain is as vivid to me as my own . . . whose faces fill the pages of my memory, faded photographs in a musty album.

Strangers, children I cradle in my arms.

Strangers, parents and grandparents of strangers, frightened, in pain, eyes focused on something far away, and I embrace them in my care.

Lives, now intertwined with mine.

Seventeen

Mrs. Travita lives down the street from me. Her husband died last year, and now she lives alone in a small brown house where the curtains are always drawn. Neighbors come during the day and sit with her. They fix her canned soup and remind her to take her medicine.

She used to talk to us in her thick Eastern European accent about her family in Yugoslavia back when it still was Yugoslavia, before we all became eyewitnesses to the atrocities.

Last week the neighbor called us because Mrs. Travita was having trouble breathing. I found her in her back bedroom, lying in bed, her hands, arthritic and knotted, pressing the covers hard against her face.

I sat beside her. "Mrs. Travita," I said to her. "It's Pat. Tell me how you're feeling."

She looked at me, her brown eyes milky, her gaze unfocused. "I'm cold," she said.

Becky spread another blanket over her, and I reached for her hand to check her pulse. It was strong and regular. Her heart was sound. "Your neighbor said that you were having some shortness of breath," I said to her.

"What?" she asked, perhaps confused by my description.

"Trouble breathing," I explained, placing my hand on my own chest.

"Yes." She nodded. "I could not breathe well."

"Is it better now?" I asked. Her respirations appeared normal.

"Yes," she said. "I am just so cold."

Joe and Mac and Maurice were waiting in the narrow hallway with the gurney. "We'll take you to see the doctor," I told her.

"I have to go to the bathroom first," she said.

Becky and I helped her up from the bed and walked her slowly to the bathroom adjoining her bedroom. I held her against me while Becky pulled down her pants, then I eased her slowly down to the toilet.

"Would you like to be alone?" I asked her.

"No," she quickly answered, reaching for my hand.

"All right," I told her. "We're right here." Becky handed her toilet paper.

We retraced our steps from the bathroom to her bed. Her respirations had increased. "Rest here for a minute," I said, covering her. "Then we'll move you to the gurney."

"I'm cold," she said.

"It's all right," I said, tucking the covers around her.

"No, it's not," she said to me, strength and anger in her voice. "It's not all right."

No. It wasn't all right.

She wasn't all right.

Her husband was dead and her country was gone.

"I'm sorry," I told her. "No, it's really not all right, is it?"

She shook her head. "No."

She cried when we moved her from her house to the ambulance.

It was a gentle ride to the hospital. We left her there and the doctor examined her and found nothing wrong, and the neighbor brought her home and fixed her soup and gave her a pill and a glass of water. And Mrs. Travita went back to bed.

I think of her some mornings when I awaken, when dawn's golden rays of sunlight reach into my house, warming and illuminating the corners of each room, and I know that a new dawn is within me as well as in the day.

I think of her sometimes.

And wish her peace.

Peace. When she rejoins her husband in the eternal country that belongs to us all.

The accident was reported, "Single vehicle into a field. Vehicle upright. Patient still in vehicle."

We traveled south on Route 20 on a blustery, stormy spring day. Sally was with me in the back. Kirk and Joe were up front.

"Fasten your seat belt," I reminded her.

"You think it's going to be serious?" she asked, buckling herself in.

"I don't think so," I responded. "Sounds like the driver just missed the turn there."

Kirk slowed and turned right on 611.

"They're probably not trapped," I continued. "Probably just waiting for us to get there."

But I was wrong.

I saw the car in the field. "Medic 292 on the scene," Joe reported to Orange Dispatch. The fire engine was just ahead of us.

The rain hit me in the face when I got off the ambulance. I saw several broken fence posts lying on the ground as I approached the car.

"I think he's got some broken ribs," Scott said. He was throwing a tarp on the hood of the car to keep the driving rain off the patient. Both the front window and the driver's window were out.

I wiped the rain off my face and started to lean into the car to check on the driver. But between the driver and me was . . . a fence post.

I called to Joe. "See if you can get in on the other side," I asked. Then I looked above the post and into the car. "Sir," I said, "can you hear me okay?"

"Yes, I can hear you," he responded. "Please get me out of here."

"Can you believe it?" Scott said. He was standing behind me. "Some luck. What do you think, Pat? Take the door off?"

I stepped back and took a good look. The eight-foot section of fence post had somehow been propelled into the car under the dash, then driven all the way to the roof of the car.

The young man's head was resting on the post.

I turned back to Scott. "Yeah," I nodded. "Let's take off the door."

I walked around to the passenger side. Joe had the door open and I crawled inside. There was no way to get him out this side. His arm was wedged between the steering wheel and the post.

I took his right hand and felt for a pulse. "What's your name?" I asked him.

"John," he said. "I'm really having trouble breathing." His respirations were very shallow. "My side hurts so bad. You gotta get me out."

His pulse was good and strong. I reached across him to check his ribs. I'd barely touched them when he screamed.

"John," I said, "I'm sorry."

Joe passed the portable oxygen in to me. "I'm going to put you on some oxygen," I explained. "It'll help."

"Will it make the pain go away?" he asked me.

"It'll help get you through this until we get you out," I told him.

Scott reached inside with a sheet to cover John's head.

"They're going to take the door off now," I explained to him, "so we can get you out."

Scott and Bruce got the door off quickly and we were able to move him out of the car. Inside the ambulance, we removed his clothes and started an IV.

I leaned over him, listening through my stethoscope to the sounds of his breathing. I could feel his shallow breaths against my face and I could smell the alcohol.

"I think we've got a pneumothorax," I told Sally. His chest sounds were diminished on the left side, and I felt the subcutaneous emphysema "Rice Krispies."

We hurried toward Mary Washington Hospital.

"John," I asked, "how're you feeling?"

"I'm so scared," he said softly.

I reached for his hand. "Take easy breaths," I told him. "Concentrate on your breathing."

Sally leaned forward to take his blood pressure.

"You'll never guess what I was doing," he said, "before this happened."

"What?" Sally asked, wrapping the cuff around his arm.

"I was at my friend's house," he said, "celebrating."

"Celebrating what?" Sally asked.

"I was in traffic court today," he said, "and it didn't go as bad as I thought it would. Shit," he muttered. "I thought it was my lucky day."

Sally and I glanced at each other.

If the fence post had entered his car a scant two inches to the left of where it did and followed the same angle, it would have taken his head off.

"My lucky day," he moaned, "and look at me now."

"Okay," Dave said, sounding, as always, a little out of breath with excitement. "It's done."

He no longer needed to identify himself over the phone.

"The ambulance is there?" I asked.

"Not quite, but it should be out of customs by the middle of August," he said. "That's when I'd like to set up the training. Does that suit you?"

"Just name the date," I told him.

"We're shooting for the middle of August. You'll be going with Claudia Huddleston and Glen Mayhew. They're from the College of Health Sciences here."

"I think that will work fine," I told him. "David leaves for the Peace Corps August fourth. He and Matt and a good friend of theirs have read Kerouac's book *On the Road*, and they're seeing a chunk of America this summer. But they're supposed to be in Salem by the middle of July."

"Good book," he said.

"I know," I agreed. "I told them I was envious."

"Don't complain," he told me. "You get to go to Mexico."

"Oh, I'm not," I assured him. "It's just that I know the language here."

"Kathy Price says not to worry. She doesn't know Spanish, either. She insists that anything she wants to say, she can say with her eyes. She told me to tell you it would be okay."

"Well," I told him, "I'm afraid it will have to be."

June 29, 1992, another Monday morning.

Another phone call . . .

"Daddy's in the hospital," my mother said. "They think he's had another heart attack."

"You'll stay at Jenny's for a few days, until band camp starts," I told Jennifer. "I'll call you tonight after I see Papa."

"Mom," she asked hesitantly, "is he going to die?"

I put my arms around her and held her close to me. "I hope not, Jennifer," I whispered.

Again, I drove to Salem.

I saw him briefly that night.

"Hey, Doc," he greeted me. His voice was weak, raspy.

"Hi, Daddy," I said. I leaned over the side of the hospital bed and kissed him firmly on the cheek. His skin against my lips was cool. "That kiss was for Jennifer, too," I told him. "She sends her love."

"Tell Rosebud I love her," he said.

My mother took his hand in hers. "We can't stay long, Al."

"It's all right," he said. "I'm probably not very good company tonight."

"You're good company for me," I said.

"Ah, Doc," he asked, "what do you know? You're just a kid."

I smiled at him. "Not hardly."

"You're my kid," he said. "Speaking of kids," he asked, "have you heard from my grandsons?"

"No," I told him. "They're probably somewhere in South Dakota by now."

"Well, let them finish their trip," he said.

He closed his eyes then.

"He's so tired," my mother said. "We need to let him sleep."

I nodded. "I know."

I reached for his hand and felt his pulse, felt the irregularity of it. I watched the monitor screen above his bed, saw the PVCs interrupt the normal rhythm of his heart. He had two IVs, one, a nitro drip, the second, lidocaine.

I knew too much, I thought to myself.

Too much.

And not nearly enough.

Oakey had left us some soup. I heated it and fixed a fruit salad. We sat down at the table, across from each other, as always.

I reached for her hands.

"Dear Lord," I prayed, "make us thankful for these and all our blessings. Please be with Daddy tonight. And with David and Matt and Jennifer. Amen."

I gave her hands a squeeze before I let go. "Now, eat something," I told her.

"What are we going to do?" she asked.

"About what, Mama?"

"About David and Matt?" she said.

140

"I don't know," I told her, shaking my head. "Let's get some sleep and then talk about it tomorrow. A very wise man taught me that," I said.

She smiled at me. "But you didn't think he was very wise then."

"Of course I didn't," I agreed. "He was my father."

I called Jennifer. "Papa sends his love," I told her.

"Jenny and I are making him a card," she said.

"Oh, he'll love that. I really miss you."

"Miss you too. Mom."

I walked into my parents' bedroom. Mama was getting her clothes ready for the next morning.

"You okay?" I asked, then sighed deeply, shaking my head. "What a stupid question."

"Come here," she said, sitting down on the bed.

I sat next to her.

"I'm so glad you're here," she told me.

"So am I," I told her. "You know there's no place else for me to be, other than here."

"I know," she nodded. "I'm just so glad that we are good friends, too."

"We're lucky, Mama," I said, putting my arms around her.

She'd lost weight, and she felt so small in my arms and so fragile. As she leaned against me I could feel her trembling.

All anyone really wants, after all, is for someone to put their arms around them and tell them everything is going to be okay.

I thought of those I have held, those I've wrapped my arms around.

I thought of Lisa and Tyler.

Of Gladys, with her drunken fears and her life, measured only in losses.

The child, Jennifer, who lost her mother on that cold Christmas night. The Cabbage Patch dolls I pulled from the wreckage. And her outstretched arms.

Jenny. Finding her safe in the school bus accident.

The mother of the children who perished in the Easter Sunday house fire. My arms around her, holding her tightly, feeling helpless against the sound of her cries.

The little girl, lost in the woods, searching for her and finding her. Her tiny hand holding mine.

Jesse.

And I thought of my own, David and Matt and Jennifer, of holding them, of wiping away their tears, chasing away their nightmares, and telling them, "It's going to be okay."

"I love you, Mama," I said to her.

Her crying had stopped. She remained there in my arms, leaning against me, and I against her.

We stayed at the hospital most of the next day.

Visiting hours in the Cardiac Care Unit were limited, and we only got to visit him for fifteen minutes every four hours, and most of the time we were with him, he was asleep.

"His heart is severely damaged," the doctor told us. "Every hour is a blessing and a positive step."

"What does that mean?" my mother asked.

"Well," he said, leaning forward in his chair, "the first heart attacks he had in 1989 were very bad. We couldn't even do a bypass. His collateral circulation has helped him through the past couple of years. But now this one seems to be a little worse than the others, and now there is an area of inactivity and a certain danger of blood clots forming."

We sat in his office, late in the afternoon, on the third floor of the hospital. I gazed out the window, west toward the distant mountains where storm-cloud shadows stretched out across the trees like black cats sleeping.

"He doesn't think we should let his grandsons know," I said, my eyes still fixed on the mountains. "What do you think?" I asked.

"I think you should think about calling them."

I turned toward him. "I've thought about calling them," I said. "I wondered what you thought."

He cleared his throat and looked at my mother, then at me. "The prognosis is not good," he said. "At this time, he has about a fifty-fifty chance. But he is a fighter, and on top of that he's got the best sense of humor I've ever seen in a patient. That gives him an edge."

"We have no idea how to find them," I said as we drove back home.

"I still don't know if that's the best thing to do," Mama responded.

"If it were me," I told her, "I would want to know."

"I would, too," she agreed. "But I want to do what your father wants."

"He wants them here," I said. "I know he does."

"You really think so?" she asked me.

"I do, Mama."

"They'll call us when they get to Seattle," she said. "That will probably be Friday."

"By then," I told her, "we'll know what to do."

It is somehow comforting here in this room, in this bed.

My room. It was here that I mourned James Dean, dressed for my prom, swooned over Elvis, cried into my pillow over lost loves and betrayed friendships. Here, I boxed up my belongings to go to college. From here, I began my life's journeys.

My window is open, and I hear the planes overhead approaching Roanoke's Woodrum Airport. Mickey's dog is barking, and a truck with a bad muffler roars down the hill in front of our house. In the distance, I hear sirens. I am unable to sleep, not because I hear planes instead of Canada geese, but because I feel that as long as I stay awake, I can stand watch. Asleep, I can be caught unaware. Asleep, I am vulnerable.

So I will stay awake.

It's difficult to tell the direction of the sirens. From the west, I think, out toward Interstate 81. But I can't be sure. I listen to the wail and the wigwag, and I can remember when flashing lights and sirens frightened me. When I lived in this house. When this room was mine and I slept in this bed.

Now, the sound lulls me.

It is soothing and reassuring, and it brings to mind good and caring people.

Sometime during the night, the phone rings.

I awaken and think, it's my sons.

But then I remember, it is not yet Friday.

Then I hear my mother cry.

"He's had a stroke," she says to me, hurrying to dress. "We have to go to the hospital."

I slip on my jeans and run a comb through my hair.

We are in the car in eight minutes.

It is two o'clock in the morning.

I have slept through my watch.

Eighteen

The doctor met us at the door of CCU.

"We're going to send him down for a CAT scan," he said. "We don't know if it's a clot or a rupture. We've got to find out so we can know whether or not to put him on a blood thinner."

I knew about strokes. I knew that a stroke caused by a clot could be transient. I knew that a stroke caused by a rupture could be fatal. And I knew of all the possibilities in between.

"What happened?" I asked.

"The nurse had just gone in to check on him," the doctor said. "He awakened and was talking to her. Then, in the middle of the sentence, he just stopped talking."

"Did he have a seizure?" I asked.

He shook his head. "No. I don't think so."

"Can he talk now?" I asked. "Can he move?"

"He can talk," he told us, "but he's got some paralysis on his left side."

My mother began to cry.

I took her hand.

"Can we see him?" I asked.

"Just for a moment," he said. "We're taking him down to X-ray."

His eyes were open, and when he saw us he smiled, but only with the right side of his mouth. It was a beautiful smile, just the same.

"Hi, honey," Mama said, leaning over the railing to kiss him.

He turned toward her, but his movement was awkward and his eyes seemed unfocused.

"I give you pretty flowers," he told her. "And candy."

"Yes." She nodded. "You take good care of me." She said it with so much love, I thought my heart would break. "We three love each other," she said to him.

He turned toward me. "Totally and completely," he said.

It was a clot.

They started him on heparin immediately to reduce the chances of another stroke.

We stayed there the rest of the night. I fed him ice from a plastic spoon.

Sometime during the night, he began to sing, "Oklahoma where the wind comes sweeping down the plain . . . homa . . . homa" but it faded away into a muffled cry.

Two days later, when he awoke, he looked at the nurse and called her Mom.

"Oh, Mr. Follmar," she said, "you know my name is Margaret."

But he only stared at her.

"Mr. Follmar," she said, leaning closer to him, looking into his eyes, "do you know where you are?"

"Why, I'm at home," he said, "in Norman, Oklahoma."

They took him down to X-ray for another CAT scan. The swelling in his brain had increased.

David and Matt called from Seattle on Friday night. The decision to tell them had been made.

"Hey, Mom," David exclaimed. "I've been calling you at home. I didn't know you were in Salem."

"David," I said, "Papa's in the hospital."

"Why?" he asked, and I could hear Matt's voice in the background.

I hated telling them this over the phone. But I had no choice. I knew it; so did they.

"He had another heart attack," I told him. "And then he had a stroke."

He cupped his hand over the receiver, and I knew he was telling Matt.

"We'll be home tomorrow," he said to me.

The next day was the Fourth of July, and Mama and I wore red, white, and blue to the hospital. We took Daddy a flag balloon and carried lunch in a picnic basket.

"It's a holiday," I announced when we walked into his room. "We're going to have a picnic." We served him tapioca and orange Jell-O, two of his favorites.

"Where's Rosebud?" he asked us.

"She's at band camp. She'll be back next week," I told him, "and she'll come see you then."

"That's good," he said, "because I keep telling the nurses I have this beautiful and smart granddaughter. They said they'd sure like to see her. But I told them I wanted to see her more." Then he asked us, "Are Dave and Matt at band camp, too?"

"No," Mama said, laughing. "Remember, they're on their trip out West?"

We'd talked about how to tell him — he, who'd always been so stoic, who never wanted to inconvenience anyone, who was so very independent.

He, who'd always made all his own decisions, had had this one made for him. How would we tell him? We would just do it.

"They'll be here tomorrow," I said.

He turned and looked at me. "Tomorrow?" he said. "They'll be here tomorrow?" And he began to cry.

I reached out and took his hand. "Yes," I repeated. "They'll be here tomorrow."

"Oh," he said softly. "They're coming home."

That night, Oakey picked my boys up at the airport. When Mama and I got home from the hospital, we all had a late dinner together. I gave them shirts I'd ordered for them, each with a picture of Jack Kerouac on it.

"A souvenir of your trip," I told them.

We cleared the table and moved into the living room. The curtains were open and we could see the sporadic explosion of fireworks in the night sky.

Mama told them about the paralysis. "But he's getting some feeling back," she added. "He cries easily," she said, "and he gets very confused."

"Does he look different?" Matt asked.

"A little," I admitted. "Mostly in his eyes. They're like a child's eyes, questioning, sometimes fearful. It's very hard to describe."

We were at the hospital at nine-thirty the next morning. Mama and I went in first. "Do you remember what today is?" she asked him.

He looked puzzled. "You mean the day of the week?" he asked.

"No," she said. "There are two young men here to see you."

"Well, send them in."

They walked into his room in front of me.

"Who the hell is that?" he asked.

I can't bear it, I thought to myself. He doesn't know them.

Then David started to laugh; then Matt, too. Mama still looked as stunned as I was.

"It's Jack Kerouac, Papa," David said.

"Of course," I sighed. "Your shirt."

Together, they wrapped their arms around him.

It was going to be all right.

Two days later, he was moved to a step-down unit. The next week, I went home to get Jennifer. I prepared her as best I could, but it was difficult. He was sitting in his wheelchair when we arrived.

"Rosebud," he cried, reaching out to her.

"It's okay, Jennifer," I told her.

"Yes." Daddy nodded, holding her tightly. "It's okay."

We were all together in his hospital room that day.

"While you were gone, we had a wheelchair race," Daddy told me.

"Who did?"

"Dave-boy and me," he said. "And I won."

I glanced at Mama and she nodded. "They really did," she said. "Down the main hall."

"Yeah," Matt said. "You won today, but I get to race you tomorrow, and we'll see who the champ is."

"You're on," Daddy said.

The nurse came in to check on him. "Mr. Follmar," she said, "you ready to get back into bed?"

"I think so," he told her. "I'm a little tired."

"Okay," she said. "I'll get some help and be right back."

But before she could leave the room, David walked to the wheelchair, cradled Daddy gently in his arms, and carried him to the bed.

"Whoa," the nurse said. "Isn't he too heavy for you?"

"Nah," David answered her, pulling the sheet up on Daddy. "He's been carrying me for twenty-three years. Now it's my turn to carry him."

Twenty-seven days after Daddy went into the hospital, he came home. The living room became their bedroom. Daddy slept in the hospital bed we'd ordered for him. Mama slept on the sofa. The dining room buffet was transformed into a medicine chest. A nurse came in twice a week to check on him and draw blood. The physical therapist visited on Monday, Wednesday, and Friday.

Life would never be the same.

But he was alive, and each day for him was a miracle.

On August fourth, David left for the Peace Corps. It was an early flight, and Matt drove him to the airport.

"I think it will be better this way, don't you?" he asked me.

"I think so," I agreed.

David got up before dawn that morning and went into the living room and lay down with Daddy. There, they said good-bye.

Dave Murray tracked me down.

"You leave in two weeks," he said. "Are you ready?"

"I guess," I told him.

"You are going!" my mother said emphatically.

"You certainly are," my father agreed.

"It's just that it's so soon, with David leaving and all. Are you sure you'll be all right?" I asked them.

"Of course," Mama said. "Matt doesn't have to go back to college for two weeks, and Jennifer will be here, too."

"Yeah," Daddy nodded. "What more do we need?"

"Okay," I agreed. "If you're sure, I'll go."

"It's been a while," I said to Joe. "I feel pretty rusty."

He glanced over at me and smiled. "That's why we travel in teams," he said reassuringly. "Do you have all your packing finished?" he asked.

"I don't think I'll ever finish," I said. "I've never been very good at packing."

"Take too much?" he asked, smiling.

"Whatever's not moving," I admitted. "Which means I've got everything in there but Nugget and the cat."

"And you leave day after tomorrow?"

"Yep." I nodded. "I still can't believe I'm really going."

"I can give you a ride to the airport," he offered.

I reached out and switched on the siren as we turned onto Wilderness Drive. "It's the next street over," I said. "And, thanks, I'll take you up on that ride."

I unhooked my seat belt and moved into the back of the ambulance. I opened the case containing the portable oxygen and quickly checked the liters — 1200 — and made sure there was a non-rebreathing mask inside.

"Medic 292 to Orange," I heard Joe tell the dispatcher. "We're on the scene."

"Rescue squad," I announced as I pushed open the door.

"In here," a man called to me.

Plastic covered the new beige carpet, and we followed it down the hall of the new, sparsely furnished house.

We found him in the den.

"Hi," he greeted us. "Come in," he said warmly, as if he'd invited us for dinner. "Have a seat."

"How are you feeling?" I asked, kneeling beside him. He was sitting in a recliner and did not appear to be in any distress. "My name is Pat and this is Joe. We were told that you were having chest pains." I placed my hand on his and felt for his pulse. It was about 80, a little weak, but regular. He wasn't short of breath.

"I'm Charlie Pierce," he said glancing at Joe, then back to me. "I was having some pain earlier — " he shrugged, " — but I'm fine now."

Joe set the oxygen down beside me. "Mike's bringing in the lifepack."

I nodded, then turned back to Mr. Pierce. "You were having chest pain and now you're not?" I asked.

He nodded. "That's right. I drank some Coke and burped a little and now the pain's gone."

"How old are you?"

"I'm fifty-six," he said.

"Any history of heart problems?"

"Nope," he responded. "Sometimes I have low blood sugar, but other than that, I'm fine."

Mike brought in the monitor and set it next to me on the floor.

"Tell me about the pain," I asked. "What were you doing?"

"Just sitting here," he said. "I was waiting for the furniture to arrive. We just got the house finished."

"It's beautiful," I told him.

"Well, I don't think the furniture's going to get here today. They just said it was an outside chance. But can I give you a tour, anyway?" he asked, and started to get up.

I put my hand on his arm. "No, not quite yet," I told him. "Right now, we're going to give you a little oxygen."

He shook his head. "I don't need that."

"Just until we decide what we're going to do," I told him. Joe placed the cannula on him. I reached out and unbuttoned his shirt. "Mr. Pierce, we're going to take a look at your heart."

"This really is unnecessary," he said.

"It's all a part of the red-carpet treatment," I told him.

Joe got the blood-pressure cuff and the glucometer out of the jump bag. I switched on the monitor and watched his EKG on the screen. Normal sinus rhythm. "Looks good," I told him. "Looks very good."

"See, a little Coke and a couple of burps will take care of anything," he said.

"Um-hum," I nodded, but I was not at all convinced.

"Blood pressure's 188 over 98," Joe said. Then he checked his blood sugar. "It's 52."

"Fifty-two, huh," he said. "I thought it was a little low."

"We need to take you to see me doctor," I said.

"Naah." He shook his head. "I'll just have some sugar."

"How about some more Coke?" I asked him. "Would you like for Mike to get you some Coke?"

"Sure," he agreed.

I glanced at my watch. We'd been on the scene for twenty minutes. "Mike, before you get the drink," I asked, "how 'bout calling dispatch and telling them our patient is stable and we'll advise as to transport."

"Okay," he said, turning to go.

"Do you know what your blood pressure is normally?" I asked Mr. Pierce.

"No," he answered me. "Why?"

"It's up a little," I explained. "Sometimes we do that to people," I said, smiling. "When you had the chest pain, did you feel nauseous or did you perspire?"

"Yeah." He nodded. "Actually, both. I was really sweating for a few minutes, and then I got a little nauseous. I think it was the bologna I had for lunch, though. We moved it down from the old house. Maybe it wasn't good."

"Show me where the pain was," I asked.

"Some in my chest," he told me, "but most of it was in my arms."

Mike handed him a glass of Coke.

"Cheers," he said to us before he raised the glass to his lips.

"Mr. Pierce," I said again, "I think you should go to the hospital."

"But you told me my heart looked fine."

"This is a rhythm strip," I said, pointing to the monitor. "It tells us you are in a normal rhythm," I explained. "Nothing else. You need a twelve-lead EKG to see what's going on."

He sat quietly for a few minutes, looking at the monitor. Then he looked back at me. "I feel fine now," he said.

"We'll recheck your blood sugar," I told him.

He scowled at Joe. "You're going to stick me again?"

"Yep," he answered. "Got to see if that Coke does work magic."

His blood sugar was 78.

We gave him some instant glucose. That brought it up to 110.

"There," he said. He pulled the oxygen cannula free of his face and handed it to Joe. "I'm fine."

"Mr. Pierce," I said with a sigh. "There is something wrong and you need to see a doctor to find out what it is."

"Okay," he conceded, "I'll see a doctor. The first thing Monday morning. Can you take these wires off my chest now?"

I leaned forward and unsnapped the leads. "You can take the patches off," I told him. "They're like Band-Aids." I switched off the monitor.

He stood up. "Well, come on," he said. "I want you to see my house."

"First, you'll have to sign this release," I told him. "It simply says that we offered you treatment and transportation and you refused."

He pulled a pen from his shirt pocket. "Just show me where to sign," he said. I handed him the clipboard.

"Put us in service on the scene, Mike," I asked.

His house was lovely. "My wife and I have everything here we've ever wanted," he told us as we moved from room to room. "Want to play a game of pool?" he asked Joe when we entered the family room.

"Another time, sure," he said.

I was looking out on the water. The view of the lake was breathtaking. "It's so peaceful," I commented.

"We're getting our boat next week. And a little sailboat for the grandchildren. I'm not sure what to do with that one," he said, "but we'll figure it out."

"You're a lucky man," Joe said.

"Don't I know it," he agreed.

"I do some sailing," Mike told him.

"He's even helped his father win some trophies," I added.

"Well, come on over," he said to Mike. "I can use your help."

Mike nodded. "Okay," he said. "Just give me a call."

"This is great," Mr. Pierce said. "I got me a sailing instructor."

"And Mike wasn't even on duty," I told him. "He lives nearby and just came to see if he could help."

"Must have been fate," Mr. Pierce said, laughing.

He walked us to the door then. "I wish you'd gotten to meet my wife," he said. "She should be home in just a few minutes, if you can wait."

"No," I told him. "Thank you, but we really do have to go. We'll meet her another time."

"Yes," he said, smiling broadly. "Another time."

He shook hands with Joe, then with Mike, then me. "Thank you so much," he said. To Mike, he added, "You'll be back soon."

Mike was back in six days. But not to teach sailing.

Again, he responded from his home to the scene. Only this time, he was the first one there. So it was up to him to break the glass and crawl inside.

Nineteen

Kathy met us at the airport in Cancún. She didn't have to introduce herself. I knew it was Kathy by the way she approached, grinning from ear to ear, and giving each of us a warm, friendly hug. "I can't tell you how thrilled we all are that you are here," she said. Watching her, I could understand how talking with her eyes was enough.

"Judith is bringing the car around. Come on," she said, grabbing several suitcases. "Let's go."

They gave us a quick tour as we traveled through Cancún; light from the strip of elegant hotels illuminated the night sky.

"Ah," Judith said to Kathy, "Just think of what we could do with what they make there in one week."

It wasn't until we arrived at the ferry dock in Punta Sam and Judith got out of the car that I was able to get a good look at her. She was very slender and attractive; and, as she stepped away from the car, her limp was quite prominent, as was her pain.

"Stay here, Judith," Kathy insisted. "Pat and I will get the tickets. Claudia and Glen can stay here with you."

"She's tired," Kathy said to me as we stood in line to pay for the ferry. "She can't be on her feet too long. Oh," she said, smiling broadly, "I just can't believe you're really here."

"After all Dave's told me, I feel like I've known you and Judith for a long time," I said to her. I hesitated for a moment, then continued. "You said that Judith tires easily. What about you?" I asked. "How are you doing?"

Her shoulders seemed to slump a bit. "Somehow, I feel I must have the strength of two even when I don't have enough for one. There's just so much to do."

It was after ten when we reached Isla Mujeres. The streets were narrow and noisy with nightlife. We sat in the hotel lobby for a while before going to our rooms.

"The ambulance is still in customs," Judith said. "We were hoping it would be out for your arrival, but things are still held up by — " she stopped and turned to Kathy " — what do you call it?"

"Red tape," Kathy answered her.

"Hmm, yes, red tape," Judith said. "Funny name. Anyway, we will go over on Thursday and see it. And tomorrow we'll go see the clinic here on the island."

"The classes will be taught in Cancún, won't they?" Claudia asked.

Judith nodded. "Yes, that seemed to be best, since their people needed some instruction, too. Our people will go over on the ferry. You will get set up tomorrow afternoon and then start on Tuesday."

"Judith, I should get you home," Kathy said. "It's late and it's been a long day."

"Ah, my friend," Judith said to her. "How did I ever get by without you?"

It had been a long day.

I lay in bed that night thinking of the hope we represented to these people and wondering if we could even come close to meeting their expectations. Kathy was right. There was much to be done.

I see poverty and deprivation in my little corner of Virginia, and I see people who have somehow fallen through the cracks. But there, when we minister to them, we have the best, the most modern equipment. And we have people we can call, social services, who can help us pull these people up and give them another chance.

Life, liberty, and the pursuit of happiness.

God, how blessed I am, I thought to myself in that small, hot hotel room. As the mosquitoes hummed in my ears, I fell asleep that first night on Isla Mujeres with the sheet pulled over my head, thinking of my father so far, far away.

The next morning, Kathy drove us past areas devastated in 1988 by Hurricane Gilbert.

"The funds simply ran out," she explained, "and these homes were never repaired."

When we reached the clinic, the first thing I noticed were the old trucks sitting in the driveway.

"The ambulances," Kathy said, pointing to them. On the side of each truck was written CRUZ ROJA MEXICANA DELEGATION ISLA MUJERES. Inside, we found some bandages and splints and cervical collars, little else.

"Tomorrow, you'll meet the kids who run calls on these ambulances," Kathy said. "They're so enthusiastic. They want to be better equipped. It's just the money."

"Isn't it always," Glen said.

I met the kids the next morning.

Claudia and Glen were working with the group from Cancún in the next room. They were teaching the more experienced students how to intubate.

I was teaching CPR to my students, the kids from Isla Mujeres. I soon discovered that talking with my eyes, while quite adequate for expressing my feelings, was not quite enough for teaching CPR. So Victor Manuel Media, an instructor and a member of the squad in Cancún, helped me. So did one of my students, seventeen-year-old Alex Maldonado, who spoke some English.

"Carlos wants me to tell you that he wants to help people who have accidents and are in need," Alex said, pointing across the room to his friend.

"Tell him I think that there is nothing more important he could do with his life."

The practice went well. I was learning their names: Claudia, and Aaron; shy and handsome Carlos; Julio, with the dimples; Naive, the youngest, who was only fourteen. There was little Matilde, Rolando, and Jovani; Enrique, who was always smiling; Damian, Arley, Jorge, and José Carmen.

They had entered the classroom cautious and unsure. By the end of the day, they could go through each scenario with self-assurance. We laughed together and shook hands and patted each other on the back. When our eyes met, our language was the same.

The next day we practiced patient assessment. We put cervical collars on each other and bandaged imaginary wounds. They took my pulse and I took theirs, counting, "*Uno, dos, tres, cuatro, cinco.*

. . ah — " I said " — what comes next, oh, yes — " I exclaimed "
— *seis.*"

"*Muy bien,* Pat," they shouted. "*Muy bien.*"

But it was Thursday they were waiting for.

Kathy came with us that morning to travel the twenty miles out of
Cancún to Customs.

The kids from Isla piled into their truck and led the way.

Victor drove the car from the Red Cross office in Cancún. Claudia
rode up front with him. Kathy and I were in the back.

"Will they let us all in?" I asked Kathy.

"Not to worry," she assured me, reaching over and patting my
hand. "Of course they will."

We pulled off the main road and into the customs parking lot.

And I saw the ambulance.

So did the kids from Isla.

They poured out of the truck and ran toward the chain-link fence.

"Pat," Matilde yelled to me, pointing to their ambulance.

I nodded and clapped my hands. She ran and threw her arms
around me. The others stood against the fence, leaning forward in
anticipation.

Kathy was right. They let us all in.

We took the boxes off the ambulance and went through each
one. There were uniforms, including ties and socks. There were
oxygen masks and a trauma box and air splints and padded-
board splints, and boxes and boxes of bandages. And there was a
radio. There were stethoscopes and blood-pressure cuffs and
thermometers.

Then we repacked all the boxes and put them back into the ambulance. We left the yard and they locked the gate behind us, and we
took our places at the chain-link fence for one last look, like new parents lingering at the nursery window.

"See." Kathy said pointing to it. "See what it says." On the side was
written: *Dedicated to the people of Isla Mujeres in honor of Judith
Fernandez. Julian Stanley Wise Foundation, Roanoke, Va. Donated by
Catawba-Masons Cove Rescue Squad, Salem, Va.* Beneath that was a list of
rescue squads and associations who had donated the equipment
inside.

157

"It's yours," Kathy said to Alex. "Tell the others for me. It belongs to all of you."

We had lunch with Victor that day, genuine burritos and tacos and guacamole dip, at a patio restaurant in Cancún.

"How did you get into rescue work?" I asked him.

"When I was eighteen," he said, "my friend was killed in Mexico City. I thought I would never get over it. Then one day another of my friends said to me, 'Let's go to the Red Cross office.' So I went." He smiled, remembering. "And I saw what was there and then I thought maybe I can help someone else live. And here I am."

"And you have helped people live," I said to him.

"Oh, yes." He nodded. "I have."

Victor drove us back to the Red Cross headquarters so we could prepare our rooms for the next day's class. "I'll be back in about an hour," he said. "I'll take you to Punta Sam in time for the ferry."

We'd just started working when the bells sounded. Once, twice, then three times, the signal for an emergency.

"Glen, get your tubes," one of the squad members yelled to him. "Get your tubes and come with us. It's a drowning."

Glen grabbed the endotracheal equipment and rushed out the door. "'Bye," he called back to us.

I looked over at Claudia. "It's a man's world," she said, shrugging her shoulders.

Victor returned in less than an hour. "Where's Glen?" he asked when he walked into the room.

"On a call for a drowning," Claudia said.

"I'll find out where they are," he told us. "And if they are at the hospital, we'll pick Glen up there."

The hospital was located on a busy downtown street. We saw the Cancún ambulance parked outside the main entrance, and, just inside, we found Glen. He was talking to a doctor. A young woman, dressed only in a bathing suit and shirt, was standing alone in the hallway dying. Her long, dark hair was wet and sandy.

Glen ended his conversation with the doctor and approached us.

"They were doing CPR when we got there," he said in a hushed voice. "The guy just went out too far in the water. Some bystanders pulled him in to shore and the woman — that's his wife — started CPR on him."

I looked her way again and was once more struck by her isolation.

"I think we may have saved him," Glen continued. "He's not breathing on his own yet, but we got his heart going."

I stepped away from them and approached the woman. Her eyes were fixed on the door that led to the room where they'd taken her husband. Even as I stood next to her, she was unaware of my presence until I reached out and gently touched her arm. I brushed the sand off the side of her face, and then took her hand and slowly led her to a wooden bench a short distance down the hall. I sat down beside her and took her hand in mine.

She turned to me once and opened her mouth as if to speak, then stopped, remembering, I suppose, that we would not be able to understand one another. Claudia sat down on the other side of her, and we stayed with her until the doctor came. He whispered something to her and she rose abruptly to go with him. But before she disappeared through the doorway, she turned and looked back at us.

"*Gracias*," she said, softly. "*Gracias.*"

I don't know what happened to him. Having Glen on the call with the intubation equipment certainly gave the victim a greater chance of survival. But there was no formal follow-up. We didn't even know his name.

So I don't know if he lived or died.

I do know now that grief sounds the same in any language. And sorrow looks the same in any country, on any face.

But so, too, does compassion.

And so, too, does love.

That night, I dreamed of my father.

The next day I tried to call Salem, but I couldn't get through.

I called Joe. The connection was bad, and I could barely hear him. "Please call Mama and Daddy," I asked him. "Make sure everything is okay."

I gave him the number at Red Cross headquarters and asked him to call me back after he talked to them. I waited.

"Not to worry," Kathy assured. She waited with me.

His call came forty-five minutes later.

"Things are fine," he said. There was a lot of static on the line, but I'd heard what I needed to hear.

"Tell them that when I land in Raleigh, I'm coming to Roanoke."

"You're not flying into Washington?" he asked.

"No. Can you hear me any better than I can hear you?"

"There's a lot of static," he said, and I could tell he was yelling.

"I want to see Daddy before I go home," I said. "Just tell them I'll call them from North Carolina. Okay?"

"Okay," he shouted. "How's everything going?"

"Great," I told him. "How about there? You and Tom and Mara holding down the fort?"

"Pretty good."

"Thanks for everything," I yelled to him. "See you — "

"Oh," he interrupted me. "Charlie Pierce di — "

"What?"

But there was only static. Then the line went dead.

"Everything okay?" Kathy asked me.

"Yes," I nodded, smiling at her. "Not to worry, right?"

That afternoon, the kids from Isla Mujeres gave me their wish list. It included boots and penlights and CPR patches to wear on their uniforms. And, as he had all week, Alex helped me with the language.

"The Red Cross has given me so much," he told me. "It's helped me to see what I want to do with my life. I will go to school in Merida and then go back to Isla and help my people."

Then he helped me tell them all good-bye.

That evening, Kathy took me to the southern end of the island.

It was dusk when we arrived. She parked the car near the lighthouse. "We'll walk the rest of the way," she said. "It's only about a half a mile."

"You sure you're all right?" I asked her.

"Not to worry," she said to me.

"When am I ever going to learn?" I said, laughing.

We paused in the fading light at Ixchel. "This is all that is left of the Mayan temple," Kathy said, pointing to its foundation. "Hurricane Gilbert really ravaged this place."

We continued down the narrow path that led to the cliffs, and I could hear the powerful waves crashing against the rocks below. We were high above the sea when the moon peeked out over the horizon.

We sat down on the ground there on the end of Isla Mujeres and watched that round and perfect moon slowly rise up from the dark, distant horizon and fill the night sky with radiance.

It was the most beautiful sight I had ever seen.

"You know," she said, "when the doctors tell you that you don't have long to live, you immediately begin to die."

"You didn't," I told her.

"I know," she agreed. "I've decided that what they meant to tell me was that I have this rare happy disease," she said to me above the roar of the sea. "That works better. Don't you think?"

"Yes, I do," I told her, directing my gaze away from the moon and toward her, my new friend.

Is the glass half empty, or half full?

Or is it overflowing?

We didn't say much more. Somehow, I felt that this was a private moment for Kathy, one in which she could rekindle her energies, pulling strength from the beauty and wonder of the night, continuing her healing in its afterglow.

It was late. My plane was fogged in at Raleigh, and I hadn't arrived in Roanoke until ten-thirty. Matt picked me up at the airport.

"Oh, it's good to see you," I told him.

"Yeah, Mom, we missed you. How was it?" he asked.

"It was incredible. I need to learn Spanish so I can go back," I said. "There was so much I wanted to say and couldn't."

He chuckled. "That must have been a hardship for you."

"I'm just going to ignore that, my son," I told him. "How is Papa?"

"He's doing good. He's still awfully weak, but he's better. Mom," he said, "how would you feel about my taking a semester off and staying with them for a while, until Papa is able to walk again?"

"I think that would be wonderful, Matt."

"I haven't said anything to them yet. I wanted to talk to you first."

"You're the best therapy he could get," I told him. "I'm really proud of you."

I spread the gifts out on Daddy's bed.

"An authentic Mexican blanket for you," I told him, "to keep the drafts away. And wind chimes for Mama."

"You're all the gift I need," Daddy said to me, smiling broadly.

I gave him another hug, then leaned back and looked into his eyes, still childlike, still somewhat frightened. "Well, I thought the moon over the island was the prettiest sight I'd ever seen," I told him. "But I guess I'd forgotten what a pretty sight you are."

We lingered at the table a long time the next morning, talking about events of the past week.

"You have to take me the next time you go," Jennifer said.

"I certainly will," I told her. "You know Spanish."

Later that morning, I called Dave Murray.

"¡Hola!"

"Pat?"

"Oh, Dave, it was really wonderful," I told him. "I wish you could have been there when the kids saw the ambulance. You deserved to be there, you know."

"I'll get there," he said. "It's just good to know we've got this great conspiracy of compassion going on."

"Is that what it's called?" I asked him, laughing.

"Sure," he said, "that's what I call it. People with vision who dare to skip Kitty Hawk and go directly to the moon."

"I like it," I told him. "I . . ."

"Mom," Matt called me from the living room.

I covered the receiver with my hand. "Just a minute," I called back to him.

"No, Mom, now," he said.

"Dave," I told him, "I'll have to call you back."

"Pat." This time it was Mama calling to me, and I could hear the alarm in her voice.

I am in the back of this ambulance holding my father's head over the blue plastic bucket Matt carried up from the basement.

He vomits again, and again. He's barely conscious. He's soaking wet with perspiration. He has dry heaves, and I know what the strain is doing to his heart.

Oh, Daddy, please don't die.

The siren wails around me. But it's not a friendly sound. It does not comfort me.

I hold his head over the blue plastic bucket, supporting him, cradling him. "I love you, Daddy," I whisper.

Twenty

It was the flu.

"Are you sure that's all?" I asked the doctor when he said they were going to release Daddy and let him go home.

"People with bad hearts do get the flu sometimes, you know. His EKG looks fine. We've given him Phenergan for the nausea. Really," the doctor insisted, "he's okay. He's just got the flu."

"It's hard," I said, "when I know how bad his heart is, not to think the worst."

Stay calm.
Remember, it's their emergency, not yours.
Oh, perhaps not always.

"It made me feel so much better," Daddy told me, "having you in the ambulance with me. I trust you," he said, resting his head on my shoulder for the trip home from the hospital. "You're my sweet and pretty little daughter, you know."

"And you," I told him, smoothing his gray hair back from his forehead, "are my sweet and handsome Daddy."

I am forty-eight years old, I thought to myself, and I have to get to know my father all over again. For he is not the father I knew before.

"It's funny," I said to my mother that night. "In lots of ways, he's the father I've always wanted."

"How is that?" she asked me, but I think she already knew.

"Well, you and I have always been close, you know, we've talked about everything. But Daddy just never talked with me much — at me, yes," I said, smiling, "but not with me. Oh, maybe I just watched too much Robert Young."

"No," she said. "I think he wanted to talk to you more, express his feelings. I just think it was hard for him to."

"You know what he told me today," I said to her. "When he was six years old, an airplane went over his house in Norman, Oklahoma. He said it was the first airplane he ever saw, and he stood there in the back yard yelling, 'Come back and take me with you. Come back and take me with you.' It was really wonderful. He never told me anything like that before. In fact," I admitted, "sometimes I thought he was born an adult. I just had trouble picturing him as a little boy."

"Hey, Mom," Matt said, poking his head into my room. "Sorry to interrupt you two, but Papa is asking for his sweet and pretty little daughter."

"Tell him I'm on my way."

Two days later, Jennifer and I went home to Wilderness. Having Matt there made it easier to leave, and I promised to call them every day.

"Matt," I said, standing in the driveway before we left. "It's such a wonderful thing that you're doing, taking a semester off and staying here with Nana and Papa. The hours will be long and unpredictable and you can't put it behind you at the end of the day, but I think it will leave you with at least as much if not more than you will be giving them."

"It already has, Mom," he told me.

It was after dark when we pulled into the driveway. Nugget was waiting for us at the door. There was a note from Joe on the kitchen counter. "Animals fed. Mail and paper on dining-room table. Gallon of milk in the refrigerator. Give me a call if it's not too late."

"Welcome home." Joe exclaimed when I called. "It's good to have you back."

"Thanks," I said. "I've got mixed feelings about being back, but it is nice to be home."

"How was Mexico?" he asked. "And your Dad?"

"Mexico was wonderful. I'm determined to learn Spanish and go back," I told him. "I had some really incredible experiences. But I can't begin to tell you about them now. And Daddy is doing" — I sighed, trying to find the right words — "better, I think. He had a touch of the flu over the weekend, but he's better now. Of course, having Matt there is going to make things so much better. What's been going on here?" I asked him.

"Squadwise?"

"Yeah. Just the highlights for tonight, though. I'm really tired."

"Well, we had a six-year-old who got a fishhook in his leg. There were two or three 1050s. Nobody was badly hurt. A couple of sick calls, a stroke, nothing really serious since the call for Charlie Pierce."

"Since then?" I asked. "That has been a long time. Did you think that was a serious call?"

"Pat. I'm not talking about the one we went on for Charlie Pierce. I'm talking about the other one."

"What other one?"

"Pat, he died."

He couldn't have.

"I told you when you called me from Mexico," he said. "I told you then."

"I didn't hear you," I said, as if that would make it not so, "It was a bad connection."

"I'm sorry," he said.

"I can't believe he died, Joe," I said, feeling close to tears. "What happened?"

The pain awakened him, like indigestion.

It was seven-thirty.

"I think I'll run down to the 7-Eleven and get a newspaper," he told his wife. He did that sometimes on weekends, picked up fresh dough-nuts and a *Washington Post*.

"Okay, honey," she said. "Why don't you come have lunch with us today?" she asked him. She kept their daughter's new baby during the week.

"I might," he said, sitting on the edge of the bed.

"You're not too young to have lunch with a grandmother, are you?" she asked, teasing him.

"Okay," he agreed. "I'll be there," he told her, wishing she would leave. He thought he was going to vomit.

She leaned over to kiss him good-bye. "I love you, Charlie," she said, her lips brushing his.

He listened to her move down the hall and into the living room. He thought of calling to her before she left, but he didn't. The nausea passed. He got up and started to dress. Fresh air will do me good, he thought to himself.

He got two chocolate doughnuts at the 7-Eleven and ate them in the car on his way back home. The pain worsened, and he was beginning to feel short of breath, as if he couldn't get enough air into his lungs.

He pulled into Lake of the Woods, but instead of turning left to go home, he turned right and drove the short distance to the Fire and Rescue Building.

"He probably thought someone would be there," Joe explained. "But of course, at that hour, no one was. So he called 911 from the pay phone and told the dispatcher he'd be at the Fire and Rescue Building. Problem was," Joe said, "when the crew got there, he wouldn't go to the hospital."

Kirk was the first one to the building. He helped Charlie Pierce onto the ambulance and asked him to lie down on the gurney.

"Oh, I can just sit here," he responded, sitting on the side bench.

"It will be easier to put the oxygen on you if you sit on the gurney," Kirk told him.

"I just need someone to check my blood sugar," he said. "I've been having some problems with that."

By that time, Norm was there, and Jack, and Bobby.

"We're going to need this space," Kirk said. "It will be better if you sit on the gurney."

"All right," he finally agreed.

He wouldn't let them put a mask on him, so Kirk used a nasal cannula. Norm got out the diabetic kit to check his blood sugar.

"The dispatcher said you were having some shortness of breath," Bobby said, hooking him up to the monitor. "Are you having any chest pain?"

"Just a little indigestion," he answered. "That's all. Look," he said, "you really don't need to go to all of this trouble. It's my blood sugar. It's low. I just need some sugar. That's what you people did before."

"And I guess," Joe said, "since we had been there once and he seemed to be fine, that maybe everybody thought that sugar was all he needed."

"What about his EKG?"

"Normal, just like before."

"Was he diaphoretic?"

"No. Kirk said his skin was normal. His EKG was normal. His respirations were 16. That's perfectly normal. Chest sounded clear. But his blood sugar was really low."

"Fifty-one," Kirk said to Bobby.

"What was it?" Charlie Pierce asked him.

"Fifty-one," Kirk repeated.

"See," he said, "that's it. Just give me a little sugar and I'll be fine."

"Have you eaten today?" Kirk asked him, handing him the tube of glucose.

"Two chocolate doughnuts," he answered. "You'd think that would do it, wouldn't you?"

"Sure would," Kirk said, smiling. "It would do it for me."

Charlie Pierce finished off the glucose. His blood sugar only went to 60.

"Mr. Pierce," Bobby said, "we need to take you to the hospital."

"I don't think so," he said, shaking his head. "I'll be fine."

"Mr. Pierce, you've got chest pain and you've had some shortness of breath. We can't seem to get your blood sugar up adequately," Bobby told him. "There's just a lot going on here, and I think you need to go to the hospital."

"No," he said, pulling off the nasal cannula. "I need to sign something, don't I?"

Kirk sighed and reached for the call sheet. "This says we offered you transportation to the hospital and you refused," Kirk said, pointing to the form.

Charlie Pierce signed it.

"Kirk even offered to drive him home," Joe said. "He wouldn't let him. Then Kirk asked him to call his wife as soon as he got home. But he didn't."

*

"What did he do?" I asked.

"He went back home, and finally I guess the pain got so bad, he called for help."

Less than an hour later, the call for "chest pain" was dispatched.

Mike knew the address and went directly to the scene. He rang the doorbell and tried to open the door, but it was locked. He rang the bell again and knocked hard on the door.

"Rescue squad," he yelled. "Open up."

He listened for the sound of footsteps. Nothing. He ran from door to door, but they were all locked. He knew the house. He'd had the tour. He thought he knew which room Charlie Pierce would be in, and he rushed to the window of the study and leaned close to the glass, cupping his hands against his face to block out the glare of the sun.

"Mike saw him through the window," Joe told me, his voice subdued, "sitting in that same chair he was sitting in before. The receiver was just lying on his shoulder, like it had fallen there right after he made the call."

Mike pulled his shirt off and wrapped it around his hand, then struck the glass, shattering it. He reached inside and unlocked it, raised the window, and crawled through. He could hear the sirens in the distance, and quickly ran to open the door. He left it ajar and returned to the study.

"When we got there," Joe continued, "Mike was doing CPR. We thought maybe there was a chance, because we knew he hadn't been down long. He was still warm. But his pupils were already dilated and fixed."

"I don't believe it," I told him. "He wasn't supposed to die."

"I know," he said.

"Was there any heart activity?" I asked him.

"Just idioventricular," he said, "nothing to really work with. We tried everything."

"We should have made him go to the hospital that first time," I said.

"We can't tie people up and make them go," Joe told me.

"We should be able to. Then he would still be alive."

"We can't be sure of that," he said.

"I'm really tired, Joe."

"I'm sure you are," he said. "Get some rest. We'll talk about all of this tomorrow."

I want someone to tell me that I did everything I could possibly have done to save Charlie Pierce.

You can't save them all.

I know that. But sometimes I think that we should be able to.

That's ridiculous. You know that in EMS there are only two rules. Rule number one is, people die. . . .

Jack Kelley was in my class of EMTs that graduated in May 1992. I call that class my smartest class, because Judy Gill made one hundred on the state exam, and not too many people have a perfect score. Jack came close. He made a ninety-eight.

"We're still not your favorite class, though, are we?" Jack asked me.

"Of course not," I responded. "Sally and Barbara and Kirk's class, now, that was my favorite class. There'll never be another class like that one," I said, smiling. "That was Christie's class, remember?"

"I remember, and I'm jealous," he said. "And we can't even be Grubnelednerts," he added, breaking into a grin.

"No way," I told him, shaking my head. "That spot's taken, too. You can't push people like Paul and Norm and Mac aside. Face it," I said, "you'll just have to settle for smartest."

"Ah," he complained, "that's no fun."

I really like Jack. He fits easily into the favorite class category, but I never told him that. I told him other things, though, back when his heart was broken and he was trying to pick up the pieces of his life. I worried about him then, and I told him so.

"I understand how you feel, Jack," I'd tell him. And I did understand. I loved someone, too, and that person had left. I was still trying to get through it.

We'd sit in his office sometimes and talk about being hurt and angry and bitter. Sometimes we'd laugh a little. Most of the time, though, we'd be just on the verge of tears.

"Jack," I said to him one day, "why don't you join the rescue squad?"

"Oh, Pat," he responded, "get serious."

"I am serious," I told him. "Christie's in college and Shannon is a senior. Don't you ever find yourself with a little time on your hands that you don't know what to do with?"

He shook his head. "I can't join the squad," he said.

"Why not?" I asked. "And don't tell me it's because you're afraid of blood because I've got the 'you've come a long way, baby,' award in that category."

"That's not it, Pat. Although I have to admit, I don't like blood."

"Jack," I told him, "no one likes blood."

"I don't know," he said, "I've listened to some rescue squad people who sound like they do."

"Yep," I agreed, "I can't argue with you there."

"I just can't do it now, Pat," he said. "Not now."

"Okay," I conceded. "But do you mind if I don't give up on you?"

"I'd mind if you did."

On August 19, 1992, at the age of eighty-seven, Sam Perry died.

Mr. Bow Tie, as he was lovingly called by members of the Fredericksburg, Virginia, community, had served on the volunteer rescue squad there for over fifty years, averaging close to 1,500 calls a year.

At City Hall, where Sam was a member of the City Council for thirty-seven years, Mayor Lawrence Davies ordered flags to be flown at half-staff.

We attended his funeral, which was held at the Fredericksburg Baptist Church, where Sam, a life deacon, had served as Sunday School superintendent for twenty-eight years. More than a thousand people listened to Mayor Davies as he spoke of a Good Samaritan in the community. That's what Sam was.

When asked about his volunteer service, Sam once said, "You can't live in this world by yourself. Everyone should help their neighbors."

Sam was always smiling. He told the corniest jokes any of us had ever heard. Elsie, his wife of fifty-two years, kept him in a rich supply of bow ties. We loved them all. He shook our hands and gave us hugs when we needed them the most.

Larry Haun, pastor of the Fredericksburg Baptist Church, said it best: "God loved the world through Sam."

He surely did.

I was on duty with Norm the day in September when we got the call for Mr. Sanders. "Possible stroke," the dispatcher told us.

We traveled down a long gravel driveway to get to the house. His wife was waiting for us on the front porch, her hands burrowed deep in the pockets of her apron.

"It just happened," she said, leading us into the bedroom. "We were having lunch and he just stopped and looked hard at me, and that was it."

"What do you mean?" I asked her.

"He just stopped talking."

He was lying in bed, staring up at the ceiling. I sat down beside him and took his hand. It was then that I noticed that he was crying.

"He's scared, I think," his wife said.

"Good morning, Mr. Sanders," I said to him. "My name is Pat, and this is Norm. We're here to take care of you. Do you hurt anywhere?" I asked him.

He shook his head. I felt his pulse. It was very irregular, and I guessed that he was in atrial fibrillation. That arrhythmia often proceeds a stroke.

Norm took his blood pressure. It was up just a little.

"Can you feel my hands on yours?" I asked him. He nodded.

"Squeeze my hands," I asked him. "Very good."

He could feel my hands on his feet, too, and had good strength and movement there as well.

"How is he?" his wife asked.

"He's not in any pain and he's not having any trouble breathing," I told her. "He has feeling and strength in his arms and legs. I think he's doing well."

"John," she said, leaning over him and wiping the tears from the corners of his eyes, "you're going to be fine."

We moved him gently from his bed to the ambulance. He was very frightened. I could see it in his eyes. They looked like my father's.

"Is there anything we can do to make you more comfortable?" I asked him.

He shook his head.

I took his hand. We traveled back down the gravel road and headed out to Route 3. "A neighbor will bring your wife to the hospital," I said to him, so he wouldn't be anxious because she wasn't with us.

He nodded.

Then he turned to me. He moved his hand away from mine and pointed to his mouth. "Why . . . can't . . . my . . . speak?" he asked me, slowly, deliberately, almost painfully, as if he had to search his memory for every word.

His eyes were childlike and frightened.

If I tell him, I thought to myself, will I add to his fears, or will I ease them?

"I think you've had a stroke," I told him.

"What . . . happen?"

He wanted to know more.

"Well," I began, "when you have a stroke, it's because there is a blockage in the blood vessels in a part of your brain. If that blockage is in the part of your brain that affects your memory, then you can't remember. If it's in the part of your brain," I continued, praying this was what he wanted, what he needed, "that affects your arms and legs, one side or the other, then you wouldn't be able to move. But it seems that the blockage was in the area that affects your speech."

I stopped and waited for his reaction. He sighed deeply and looked out the back window of the ambulance.

Then he turned and faced me again. He smiled. "So . . . I . . . am . . . lucky," he said, nodding vigorously.

"Yes," I agreed, looking into his eyes, still childlike but not as frightened. "I think you are," I told him, thinking of my father, "I think you are very lucky."

Twenty-One

For Jack's forty-fourth birthday, I gave him an application to the rescue squad. Three months later, he joined.

"I think I'm ready," he told me. "But, for now, just put me on as a substitute."

He was covering for Pia when the man fell off the ladder.

Norm called for ALS and I met them on the scene. They had the patient immobilized, and his arm was splinted. It was in an awkward position, and Jack was holding it to provide additional support.

"His blood pressure is really low," Norm said as I set up a line of Lactated Ringers. It was 90 over 60. The man seemed alert. Jack was talking to him in a low, calm voice, and the man was responding to Jack's questions.

"I've been a carpenter all my life," he said. "Had pretty good luck up to now. I'm sixty-seven, so I guess I can't complain."

"His arm is really bad," Norm continued, talking quietly so our patient couldn't hear. "He must have fallen on his hand. It looks like he dislocated his elbow and pushed it right through the skin. The humerus is broken, too."

I wondered how he was tolerating the pain. All of his attention was on Jack. The two of them continued to talk to each other even while I started the IV and hooked him up to the cardiac monitor. It was as if they were drawing strength from each other.

When we arrived at the hospital and moved the man into the trauma room, Jack continued to hold on to his arm. The nurse came in and took our report. We'd seen no indication of internal bleeding, and his blood pressure had come up with the fluid. His level of consciousness was very good. He seemed to be okay except for his arm.

It was time for us to go.

"Well, Henry," Jack said to him, "you take good care of yourself. I hope to see you again sometime under better circumstances."

Henry held up his good arm and reached over to shake Jack's hand.

"Thanks, partner," he said. "You really took good care of me."

Norm rode up front with Darren. Jack and I were in the back.

"It was hard to tell him good-bye," he said.

"I think it was hard for him, too," I told him, "to let you go. Do you realize what pain he must have been in?"

"Yeah." He nodded. "He was really brave."

"He was brave," I agreed. "But you made it easier for him."

"Because I held his arm?"

"That, and more, Jack."

"I've been on about ten calls," he said as we pulled away from the hospital. "Henry's arm was the worst injury I've seen. I've been on several calls for strokes and a diabetic call. Then there was the child with the bean in his nose," he continued, smiling, "and I was with Kirk the day it snowed and so many people slid into ditches. I think we went on four calls for wrecks and didn't even need a Band-Aid. But I always learn something on every call," he added.

I nodded. "I do, too. So," I asked him, "what do you think?"

"I feel like I haven't really been tested yet," he responded. "Like something big is going to happen, and I want to know I'll be able to handle it."

"Jack," I said to him, "I watched you with our patient, with Henry, and the way you talked to him, it was like the two of you were the only people here. He wasn't just a shattered arm to you. He was a person."

"It kind of felt like we were the only ones here," he admitted.

"You're going to be fine," I told him.

I leaned back in the seat and propped my feet up on the gurney, and gazed out the back window of the ambulance. We passed through the city streets of Fredericksburg and out into the county, heading home.

"This is giving me my life back" he said, startling me a little with the intensity of his words.

I shifted my gaze to him.

"We forget, sometimes, the pain of others," he continued. "We think we're the sole owners. Then, the curtain is lifted. And we see. And each time I go out on this ambulance, the curtain is lifted a little more."

It was ten-thirty on a Saturday night. I'd had a bad cold and fever most of the week, and was already in bed.

Jennifer brought me a glass of orange juice and set it on my bedside table. "Is it okay if Jenny and I stay up awhile and watch TV?" she asked me. "We'll keep it turned down low."

"That's fine, darling," I told her. "You won't keep me awake. Thank you for the orange juice."

"You're welcome, Mom," she said. "Hope you feel better."

I switched off my light, pulled the covers up to my chin, and closed my eyes.

The tones went off.

"OB call in Lake Wilderness," the dispatcher said.

There was a time I would have thrown my covers back, jumped out of bed, and rushed out on that call.

But, as Jean used to say: "To what avail?"

"We're never going to get to deliver a baby," I complained to Joe one day, finally conceding that the odds were just too stacked against us.

Back in August 1990, Sally Kelley, one of my Grubnelednerts, a member of the squad (and Jack's sister-in-law), called the squad when she went into labor and she and her husband Bob suddenly feared she wouldn't make it to the hospital in time for the birth of their son. That would have been our big chance — except that, as it turned out, there wasn't even enough time for us to get there.

I did get to cut the cord.

And so, I became reconciled to the fact that it was just not to be.

Night Team 3 was on. Phyllis, Barbara, Darren, Holly, and now Jack. He had decided it was time to go off the sub list and onto a regular duty crew.

That night, Darren had Andy covering for him. Kathy, just coming home from work, asked if she could go, too. It was a full crew. I heard Holly request directions and mark en route to the scene. I switched on my light and reached for the glass of orange juice. I was wide awake.

Nothing will happen, I thought to myself. The mother-to-be will have her bag packed and be waiting at the door. It will be another easy ride to the hospital.

"Rescue 291 is on the scene," Andy announced to dispatch.

The front door was wide open, and they could hear her yelling when they pulled into the driveway.

"Let's go," Kathy shouted, grabbing the OB kit and jumping off the ambulance. Jack was right behind her.

Her water had already broken, and when they entered the house, they found her leaning against the sofa. "It's coming," she said. "The baby's coming now." Beside her, tightly gripping her leg and crying loudly, was her three-year-old son.

Phyllis picked the boy up and carried him from the living room, talking to him, soothing him. Soon, his crying stopped. "What do you want, sweetheart?" she asked him, "a brother or a sister?"

"A sister," he said, smiling at Phyllis.

Jack and Barbara helped the mother down onto the gurney. "Squeeze my hand," Jack said to her as another contraction started.

I wish they'd say something, I thought to myself. Maybe they just forgot to mark en route to the hospital. Why don't they say something?

"It's a boy!" Holly squealed.

"It's a brother!" Phyllis said to the little boy in her arms. "Is that okay?"

"Yes," he yelled, clapping his hands.

"It's a boy," Andy announced over the radio. "It's a boy."

I threw the covers off and opened my bedroom door.

"Hey," I yelled down the hall to Jennifer and Jenny. "It's a boy!"

They just looked at each other.

I waited until I heard the crew mark back in station and I went to the phone to call them, but they beat me to it.

"I wish you'd been there," Barbara said to me.

"Me, too," I agreed. "But if it couldn't have been me, I'm glad it was you."

"My face hurts from smiling," Jack said, laughing. "I don't think I can stop."

"Congratulations," I said to all of them.

But it was Phyllis whose words I shall never forget, "Oh, Pat," she said, her voice close to breaking. "When I held the baby, I kept thinking: Last year I held Dick in my arms as he died. And now, I'm holding a brand new life."

December 22, 1992.

Jennifer and I were leaving for Salem the next morning to spend the holidays with Mama and Daddy and Matt. With David in Ecuador and Daddy ill, I knew this Christmas would be quite different from previous ones. But I also realized how lucky we all were to have one another.

Our monthly squad meeting was that night, and I'd invited our new family from Lake Wilderness for a special stork-pin presentation.

It was the beginning of Christmas vacation and schools closed early. Jennifer was wrapping presents and I was working on the agenda for the meeting.

And I was on duty.

It was around three o'clock when I heard Battlefield's tones go off. We run a lot of mutual calls with them. Many of my students came from the Battlefield squad: Jim and Becky and Frank, Gretchen and Trahn and Laura. And I have old friends there, too, Ray and Van and Nancy, Howard and Cathy and Mike.

So I listen closely when I hear their tones.

Mary Kay Mayo got off the school bus that afternoon feeling like she might be coming down with the flu. She was in the sixth grade at Lightfoot Elementary school, and at the Christmas party that day, she hadn't felt much like eating.

Cathy and Mike were out working on their farm when Mary Kay arrived home from school. When Cathy came in from the field, Mary Kay met her at the door.

"Mama, I don't want to be sick for Christmas," she said.

Cathy gave her some juice and tucked her in bed, and called her piano teacher and canceled her three o'clock lesson. Mary Kay dozed off.

She awoke a little before three and called for Cathy.

"I feel sick again," she said.

Cathy helped her into the bathroom, but Mary Kay became dizzy and slumped down onto the floor.

By then, Mike was home and Cathy called to him to help her get Mary Kay back into bed.

"Would you like to lie down in our bed?" Cathy asked her. It was closer to the bathroom.

"Yes," Mary Kay said, in a weak voice, smiling up at them. "It's a nice big bed and I can roll over."

Then her eyes closed and her breathing became labored, and she didn't respond when they called her name.

"Go get the ambulance," Cathy told Mike. "I think she's having a seizure."

The call is for seizures. A twelve-year-old with seizures.

A fever, I think to myself. A fever will bring on seizures in children. I turn back to my desk and pick up my pen.

Cathy waited for the seizure to pass. But when it stopped, so did Mary Kay's breathing. So did her heart.

"Cecilia," Cathy shouted to her older daughter. "Come help . . ."

Cathy and Cecilia began CPR.

I hear, ". . . not breathing . . . at the Mayo residence . . ." Pam is dispatching, and I can hear the pain in her voice as she tries to say the words we all must hear. "Mike's gone to get the ambulance . . . any available personnel respond . . . CPR in progress . . . CPR in progress."

I grab my jacket even before I hear Van on his portable radio tell Pam to "tone out Lake of the Woods." Even before she sets our tones, I am in the car and out of the driveway. I hear her saying it again, ". . . twelve-year-old child at the Mayo residence . . . CPR in progress . . ." I press my hand against the horn all the way to the building and the cars move out of my way. I am driving too fast, I know. I realize that I am praying.

Joe drives the ambulance because he knows the way to Mike and Cathy's house. We don't need the 911 page and grid. We head down Route 20, and my mouth is so dry I feel that no words will come if I try to talk. Outside and around us, the sirens scream. Inside, there is silence. I am suddenly aware of the tears that dampen my face.

I hear Kelly on Medic 230 mark en route from Orange. Pam gives him directions and her voice is hollow . . . for we are all friends . . . and this is too much to bear.

Howard gets there first because he lives just across the field, on the adjoining farm. Then Kelly and David. They defibrillate twice and give epinephrine, and call for Pegasus.

We arrive and I run into the house and into the bedroom, where they are doing CPR on Mary Kay. I go to Cathy, and put my arms around her and hold her. I ease her up from the chair where she is sitting and, with my foot, push aside the jump bag and the oxygen tank and the IV box to clear a way for us out of the room.

I help her to a chair in the living room. I dial the phone for her so she can arrange for her older son to get a ride home from wrestling practice. Cecilia is in the kitchen, crying. Mike's parents are there. They travelled from Congers, New York, the night before to be there for Christmas and they are not well. What must this be doing to them?

I am stricken suddenly with the thought that I don't want to do this anymore. It just hurts too much.

Mike comes into the room and tells Cathy that Mary Kay is breathing a little on her own, and that there is a heartbeat. I leave them there together and go back into the bedroom. Howard has intubated her, and Joe is doing ventilations because Mary Kay's sporadic breaths are not enough. An IV is started, and we administer Dopamine to raise her blood pressure. The ectopy continues with runs of bigeminy. We give her lidocaine, and she returns to normal sinus rhythm. We are on our knees on a bedroom floor working on a child . . .

I don't think I want to do this anymore.

"Ten minutes on Pegasus," Brook announces.

"Let's move her to the ambulance," Howard says. "Then we'll drive down to the field."

There are eight of us here in this room and we move as one. We do not fumble, nor do we get our oxygen and IV lines crossed. We move quickly and there is cadence in our steps. For we are carrying someone very precious.

I hear the whirring sound of Pegasus in the distance as we move down through the field to the landing zone. The back doors to the ambulance are opened and I see Milt there. Chief of Mine Run Fire Department, he is in charge of the landing zone. But, more than that, he is their friend, and in his face, I see a reflection of my own.

I wonder if we have all grown tired.

We carry her through the tall grass down to the helicopter and I linger there, briefly. I touch her dark hair once more, and caress the soft skin of her forehead. Her eyes, half open, show no recognition, no sign of having felt my touch.

We walk back through the field and turn and watch as Pegasus lifts off. The wind from the helicopter turns the grass into oceanic billows, waves left behind in its wake. Pegasus rises into the air and heads southwest toward Charlottesville.

And it's over.

That night, I awarded stork pins in a celebration of life.

The next day, I traveled to Salem with Jennifer to be with my family for a celebration of Christmas and family.

Mary Kay lay in a coma.

On Christmas Day, I called Terry. I knew she'd be working in dispatch. Terry also ran with Battlefield and was Mike and Cathy's friend.

"Orange County Sheriff's Department," she answered.

"Hi, Terry," I said to her. "Merry Christmas."

"Pat, Merry Christmas. Are you home?"

"No," I told her. "I'm still in Salem. We'll be coming home tomorrow. I just wanted to know how Mary Kay is."

"She's still in a coma," Terry said.

"Do they have any idea what happened to her?"

"Evidently, she had some very rare heart problem, like extra electrical wiring. Nothing could have prevented what happened."

"Mike and Cathy," I said, "how are they?"

"As well as can be expected, but no one is doing very well, really. No one. You know," she said, "the Sunday before this happened, Mary Kay played Mary in the Christmas program at church. I keep remembering that, the way she looked."

"Terry," I asked. "What's the prognosis?"

"It doesn't look good," she said, "not good at all."

The next day, Jennifer and I told Mama and Daddy and Matt goodbye. I held each of them a little closer to me before letting go.

I never really believed that Mary Kay would die. I don't think any of us did. We had a prayer chain and a telephone chain and I don't remember a time when the people of this county came together the way they did when Mary Kay Mayo lay in a coma.

On December twenty-seventh, the doctors thought there was some movement in her legs and perhaps the EEG showed something. We were hopeful.

On December twenty-eighth, there was nothing.

And on December twenty-ninth, my birthday, Mary Kay died.

Her funeral was held on Thursday, December 31, at Antioch Baptist Church near the Mayos' home, and all of us who straggled so to save her life sat together in a section reserved for rescue-squad members. Rev. Terry Green spoke to us about how special children are to Jesus and how God loves and cares for us all.

"Things happen," he said to the crowded sanctuary, "and we have no explanation for them. God does not cause bad things to happen. He is there to comfort us when they do.

"Mary Kay touched all our lives," he continued. "Her family, her friends, her church, and her community are richer because of Mary Kay. She did more to comfort and to teach and to show God's love in her twelve short years than so many other people do in a lifetime."

We carried the flowers out to the cemetery that adjoined the church-yard and placed them at the gravesite. On that cloudless, warm, and radiant winter afternoon, we stood in a circle around our friends and listened to the final prayers for the child who had touched us all.

Twenty-Two

We were a ragtag bunch, small on experience and big on dreams, most of us carryovers from the sixties, when dreams in America were too costly. In 1974, when I met Bill Clinton, embers still smoldered in Vietnam. Watergate continued to dominate the news. We were a nation desperately in need of heroes.

I met Bill at a meeting of the Washington County Democrats back in February 1974. He was sitting four rows behind me. I was relatively new to Arkansas and had never heard of Bill Clinton; but then, few people had.

Toward the end of the meeting, he was introduced. "I'm running for Congress," the twenty-seven-year-old University of Arkansas law professor told the group of Democrats. "I can beat John Paul Hammerschmidt, but I need your help to do it."

We were there the next week to sweep out the old house on North College Avenue, the Clinton for Congress Headquarters.

David was in kindergarten and Matt in preschool, and each morning, after I took them to school, I would go straight to headquarters. Barbara Rudolph and I shared an office in what had been the dining room of the old house. Cindy sat at the desk out front, in the reception area. The hall led to a bathroom and two back rooms. One was Bill's office. The other was a press room with a TV, bookshelves, more telephones, and a copier. There was always coffee brewing in the kitchen.

Barbara and I traveled through the twenty-one counties in the third congressional district, distributing bumper stickers and brochures to each local coordinator. We arranged appearances for him at wine festivals and poultry festivals and picnics and church functions. We'd drive through the Ozarks and down the mountain into Alma and Sebastian County, then turn eastward across to Pope, turn north to Searcy, and then head back to Fayetteville.

Bill made us believe that things could be better for everyone. He spoke of social justice and a fair tax system, quality education and a national health program. Crowds around the district were increasing, and the early trickle of volunteers through campaign headquarters was growing into a steady stream. From students to senior citizens, they came. And Bill had gained the attention of Governor Dale Bumpers and Congressman David Pryor, both of whom would become United States senators.

Hillary Rodham joined us in October, and we welcomed her on board. She'd traveled from Washington and her job as a staff member on the House Judiciary Committee to help pull things together. We knew Bill could beat Hammerschmidt if we all worked hard enough, and we worked nonstop. The last weeks of the campaign were grueling.

On November 5, 1974, we were up before dawn. We worked the polls and we voted for the man who promised hope. And we waited.

Bill came within a hair of beating John Paul Hammerschmidt, earning 48.2 percent of the vote and winning thirteen of the twenty-one counties. The National Committee for an Effective Congress referred to Bill's race for the House as "the most impressive grass-roots effort in the country."

That was little consolation for us.

But, even in defeat, we all knew it wasn't over. It was far from over.

We wrote occasionally, a congratulatory card when he and Hillary were married and when he became Arkansas's governor, another at Chelsea's birth, and when he declared his candidacy for President. We heard from them when Jennifer was born.

"How way leads on to way," Robert Frost wrote in "The Road Not Taken." And so it is. The years pass and moments are forgotten, and faces and places are not so clearly in focus. But, dreams are constant. Hope endures.

At first I thought it was just a rumor. Bill and Hillary and Chelsea and the Gores coming to Culpeper? But there it was, on the front page of the *Culpeper Star Exponent*, and on the nightly news.

So, I called my friend Wanda Gardner.

"Do you need any more units for the seventeenth?" I asked her.

"Maybe," she said. "I'm teaching a class that day, and I'm not even going to be there."

"Well, if you need another ALS unit, we'll be glad to provide one."

"Thanks," she responded. "We're going to have a meeting next week, and I'll let you know."

"Wanda," I began. "I've got to tell you. I have an ulterior motive. I knew them, Bill and Hillary, a long time ago. I'd really love to see them one more time before he's sworn in."

She laughed. "You know," she said, "this area wasn't real strong for Clinton, so it might be nice to have someone here who is so gung ho. I really appreciate your offer. I haven't made any definite plans yet. That's, what, three weeks away?"

"Yeah."

"There are supposed to be close to 5,000 people here that day, and I do know we can always use another ALS unit."

"Just give me a call," I said with fingers crossed.

She called me a week later. "We're going to station you at the Culpeper Baptist Church," Wanda said. "Clinton will be there for the eleven o'clock service and that's where most of the crowd will be, outside the church."

"You want us at the church?"

"Yeah," she said. "Is that okay?"

"Wanda, that's perfect!" I told her.

"I talked to Billy and Tim, and they're going to bring a unit from Richardsville. I'm going to put all of you close to the church to handle the crowds there, since you don't know the Culpeper streets like our people do. Our units will be on either end of town. You will handle any ALS calls in the crowd."

I couldn't believe it!

I wrote Bill and Hillary and told them. "I'll be in Culpeper," my letter said, "at the church. I'll be near the LAKE OF THE WOODS VOLUNTEER RESCUE SQUAD ambulance. I hope I get to see you."

All that week, a cold rain fell.

But on Sunday morning, January seventeenth, the sun rose into a sky of solid blue.

Sally drove and I rode up front with her. Jack and Joe were in the back. "I'm so excited," Sally said as we pulled into Culpeper.

"Sally, I'm glad you're here," I told her. "I don't think the guys could muster enough enthusiasm. I don't even think that Jack voted for him," I said, loud enough for him to hear me.

"I didn't," he admitted. "But there was no way I was going to miss seeing you see him. I brought my camera along just for that."

"Okay," I nodded. "I hope you have lots of film."

"Gosh, it's been so long since I've seen them," I said to Sally. "Almost twenty years. We're different in many ways, but in the ways that brought us all together, I know we're still the same."

She glanced over at me. "You really think we're going to get to see them, don't you?"

"I do," I said. "I really believe it. And I think we'll get to talk to them, too. Things will just work out," I told her.

"I know they will."

We turned north on Main Street at eight o'clock. Flags lined every street. We drove beneath a sign that read WELCOME TO CULPEPER, PRESIDENT-ELECT BILL CLINTON. It was only eight, but crowds were already forming on street corners.

We picked up our radio and map from the Culpeper Rescue Squad building and worked our way through the crowds and the TV vans to our position on the corner of Blue Ridge and Scanlon. The church was at the bottom of the hill.

"It's only nine o'clock," Joe said. "Why don't we walk around some?"

"We'll just lock up the ambulance," I told him. "I have the radio. We'll hear them call if they need us."

"They won't need us," Jack said. "I've got all of this film." I smiled at him. "I sure hope you're right."

We milled through the crowd surrounding the church. There were small groups of demonstrators — environmentalists, pro-life, and pro-choice — and secret-service personnel with tiny plastic wires snaking up from their heavy coats into their ears. A woman handed me a small American flag.

"What a wonderful day," she said to me before she continued through the crowd.

"Oh, yes," I agreed.

Sweet strains of organ music flowed from the church through the outside speakers. There was promise in the crisp morning air.

At ten-thirty, the police asked us to move behind the ropes. We were across from the church and up nearly half a block, but from where we stood we could see across West to Main Street. We'd see the bus caravan when it passed. Sally stood beside me. Jack and Joe were behind us.

"The buses . . ." someone shouted. "He's coming!"

I stood on the curb, pushed forward by the crowds behind me, holding tightly to the rope with one hand, to my flag with the other. We watched the buses two blocks up, saw them pass down Main, and counted the seconds until we saw the first one pull up to the church.

There he was, sitting in the front seat across from the driver, a cup of coffee in his hand, jotting down some last minute notes . . . and it was nineteen years ago . . . traveling through the mountains of northwest Arkansas on a campaign trail held together by a shoestring budget and dreams of a brighter tomorrow. I waved my flag. Tears stung my eyes.

"Bill . . . Bill," the people chanted as he stepped off the bus. "Over here," came the shouts from every corner. He looked into the crowd and waved. Then he walked with Hillary and Chelsea down the sidewalk to the church.

I heard "Culpeper Dispatch to EMS Command," and pulled my radio from my pocket and raised it to my ear.

"This is Command," Tim acknowledged. "Go ahead."

"I just got a call for chest pains on West Street. What unit do you want to respond to it?"

"Send Lake of the Woods," he said. "They're closest."

I turned to Sally and Joe and Jack. "We've got a call," I yelled to them above the noise of the crowd.

We found our patient lying on the ground. Someone in the crowd had covered her with a blanket.

"Tell me where it hurts," I asked, kneeling over her, shielding the sun from her eyes.

"Here," she said, her fist clenched and pressed against the middle of her chest.

"Sharp? Dull?" I asked.

"Sharp," she said. "I think it's my hernia. I didn't take my medicine this morning after I ate breakfast." She smiled broadly. "I think I was just too excited."

I returned her smiled. "I understand."

She sat up and Joe helped her to the gurney and he and Jack lifted it onto the ambulance. Joe drove, easing the ambulance carefully through the congested street. I hooked her up to the monitor: normal sinus rhythm. She told us she was fifty-nine years old and had no medical history other than the hernia. The pain had lessened.

"I feel so silly," she confessed as Sally wrapped the blood-pressure cuff around her arm. "It happened when I saw the bus," she admitted. "I just got so excited. I really think that's what happened to me. Just excitement."

"I don't think it's at all silly," I told her. "Believe me," I said, "if I had a hernia, mine would act up, too."

"I'm not used to being this close to a hospital," Joe said as we pulled away from the loading dock.

"I know," Sally agreed. "I barely had time to take her blood pressure."

"But the good part is that we can get back fast," I told them. We turned back onto Blue Ridge at 11:20.

Jack grinned at me. "I'll get my camera ready."

We took our places behind the ropes and listened to Rev. Herbert Browning's sermon over the loudspeakers. He spoke of Daniel in the lion's den and his trust in God even in the face of opposition. "Not living our convictions," he said, "is the only thing that costs more than living them."

"Pat," Sally whispered, tugging on the back of my jacket. "Look at that woman."

I turned to her. "Where?"

"They just went by us," she said. "She's across the street now."

I looked up and saw the couple, the man and woman. His arm was around her in what initially appeared to be nothing more than a loving gesture. But as I watched them more closely, it became evident that he was helping to support her as she walked. We stepped over the ropes and started in their direction just as the woman stumbled.

She could barely stand. We gently eased her down to the ground while Jack went for the ambulance. She was cold and very diaphoretic. Her respirations were rapid and labored.

"She'd taken three of her nitro pills," her husband said, "and it didn't help. She's in so much pain. We saw the ambulance there and we were going for help."

When Jack arrived, we quickly moved her onto the unit. Her pulse was very weak, and the monitor showed first-degree heart block. We put her on oxygen and I recorded her vitals on the call sheet, and the time, 11:50.

Her level of consciousness improved a little with the oxygen. Her blood pressure was high, and her respirations were still labored. We were at the hospital in four minutes.

"She's in bad shape," the nurse told us as we were getting clean sheets for the gurney. "With her history, she should never have been out there for so long. It's a good thing you all were there, to get her here so quickly."

"How's our first patient?" Joe asked.

"She's going to be fine," the nurse replied, smiling. "She did a good self-diagnosis. Hernia and excitement."

It was 12:11 when we turned back down Blue Ridge.

"Church probably ran a little late, don't you think?" I said to Sally.

"I'm sure it did," she agreed.

Joe backed into our parking space on Scanlon.

I stepped off the ambulance.

And then I saw that the crowd had dispersed and the people who had stood behind the ropes with us were milling around in the street. One of the women looked up as I approached them, saw me, and shouted. "You should have been here. Bill and Hillary and Al Gore came right over to where we were standing. They shook our hands and talked to us. It was wonderful" — she continued to shout — "wonderful!"

I thought to myself, You don't know them well enough to call them Bill and Hillary. I turned around and walked back to the ambulance. "I'm going to be all right," I said to Sally and Joe and Jack. "Just give me a few minutes."

I still do not know why my disappointment was so overwhelming and so painful. I do know that I was too sure it would happen. Perhaps I thought that I deserved that moment — because I was a part of that ragtag bunch that first believed in Bill Clinton, that inner circle that planted the initial seeds when the land was cold and the ground was barren, knowing and believing that spring would come — and finally, wanting desperately to share in that moment of fruition.

But they were gone.

My moment had passed.

I dried my eyes and got off the ambulance and walked back to the others. "It's okay, guys," I told the crew.

"No, it's not," Sally disagreed. "I really wanted to meet them."

I gave her a hug. "Next time," I said. "There has to be a next time."

Joe rested his arm on my shoulder. "Pat," he began, "when I was nine years old I got a new sled for Christmas. It was a beauty. I was out sleighriding with some of my friends and one of them got hurt. Something happened and he was cut on the blades of the sled."

"Joe," I said, puzzled at his remarks, "where is this going?"

"You'll see," he said, smiling. "Just hold on. Anyway," he continued, "I ran over to him and tried to stop the bleeding and then I stayed with him until his mother came. And then, when I went back for my sled, it was gone."

"Gone?" I asked. "You mean somebody took it?"

"Yep," he answered me. "Somebody took it."

I smiled up at him. "You're a good friend, Joe Broderick," I told him. "And your analogies aren't bad, either. Thanks."

"Nothing to thank me for," he said. "I just happened to think of that and thought you might like to hear it."

"Command to all rescue units," Tim announced. "Command is now terminated. Please acknowledge."

"Medic 292 acknowledges," I reported when our turn came. "Medic 292 is returning to station."

We started toward the ambulance and I turned around to take one last look at the church. A woman was walking toward me. A young boy was holding her hand.

"Pat," she said, drawing closer, "I can't go on any longer."

"Theresa?" I said, suddenly recognizing her. An acquaintance from the Lake, she'd moved away several years before. "What's wrong?" I asked her. She was pale and looked as if she were about to faint.

"I'm so sick," she said as Sally and Jack helped her onto the ambulance. I took the boy's hand and Joe opened the side door for us. I let him sit on the bench so he would be with Theresa. He was trying to blink back his tears.

"It's okay, Paul," she comforted him. "Mama's fine." She reached out and touched his face, wiping away his tears. Then she looked at me and smiled. "I feel pretty embarrassed," she said. "I think I may just have a bad case of the flu, but I couldn't walk any further." She lay her head back and closed her eyes, then opened them and turned to her son.

"But, we did it, Paul, didn't we! We did it!"

The boy nodded then and smiled a radiant smile.

Twelve-year-old Paul Hull had portrayed Bill Clinton in the Culpeper Middle School mock election in November. He'd debated two other youngsters who represented George Bush and Ross Perot. And he'd won! In his middle school, in an overwhelmingly Republican county, the election results were: Clinton, 34 percent; Perot, 30 percent; and Bush, 26 percent.

So, when Paul Hull read that Bill Clinton was coming to town, he begged his mother, "Can we go, Mom? Please?" He just wanted to shake Clinton's hand.

Theresa got sick the night of January sixteenth, very sick. But the next morning there was no one else to take Paul, so she took two aspirin to keep her fever down, and at seven o'clock they headed for the Culpeper Baptist Church.

"You ever going to wash that hand, Paul?" she asked her son.

"I don't think so," he responded. His tears had dried and his eyes were wide with excitement, remembering.

"Bill Clinton shook Paul's hand," Theresa said, smiling. "I held on till then," she said, "because I didn't want to ruin Paul's day. I didn't know what I was going to do. Then I saw you all," she said, smiling up at Jack and Sally and me, "old friends, and I knew I'd be okay. And I knew Paul would be okay, too."

So the day ended with one last trip to Culpeper Memorial Hospital in the company of a twelve-year-old boy whose dream had come true. He'd shaken hands with his hero, and mine, Bill Clinton.

Twenty-Three

Up until I was two years old, while my father was overseas in the Marine Corps, my mother and I lived with my grandparents in Roanoke, Virginia, in a comfortable two-story brick house on Mt. Vernon Road.

Running perpendicular to Mt. Vernon was Terrace Road, and my grandfather had a vegetable garden near the corner where the roads met. It was a nice-sized garden, roughly fifty by a hundred feet, and he planted corn and green beans and tomatoes and three kinds of peas and two kinds of squash, and onions and potatoes and carrots.

In the winter months, he would till and mulch the soil. In the spring, he'd plant the seeds and young seedlings, and in the summer and early fall, he'd pick bushels of fresh, sweet-smelling vegetables that my mother and grandmother would cook and can. So we spent a lot of time on the corner where Mt. Vernon and Terrace Roads met.

A neighbor of theirs who lived with his wife on Terrace Road had a flower garden. His specialties were roses and petunias, and often, as he was tending his flowers, he would wave across to Granddaddy in his vegetable garden. When my mother took me for walks, first in my carriage, later in my stroller, we would pass by the white brick house that belonged to the man and his wife. My mother would stop and admire the roses and petunias and the pink and white flowering dogwood trees.

My mother and I moved away from Mt. Vernon Avenue to Salem when my father came home, but we visited every weekend, and when I grew older, I'd spend several weeks there during the summer when my cousins came to visit. We'd drink lemonade and play canasta on the front porch and walk down Mt. Vernon and across Terrace to Lakewood Park, where we'd feed biscuits to the ducks.

We'd walk by the white brick house. But, being young and not caring a whole lot about flowers or grownups, we'd pay little attention to the man in the yard or to the roses and petunias that he tended.

So I don't remember him at all.

My mother remembers very little about him. It wasn't until I began gathering information on the history of volunteer rescue squads that we came to know whose house it was, who cared for the flowers and waved to my grandfather.

It was Julian Stanley Wise.

I thought about that for a long time, the fact that he lived so close to us. Granddaddy probably gave him fresh vegetables, and maybe he gave Granddaddy cut roses to take home to my grandmother. That certainly would have been typical of both of them.

Because I now know that people are comprised of so much electrical energy, I sometimes wonder, strange as it seems, if he might have given off a spark one summer evening when my mother and I passed by.

I wonder.

In the movie *Dead Poets Society*, Robin Williams plays an English teacher who encourages his students to turn their lives into something extraordinary. He says to them, quoting from Whitman:

The powerful play goes on and you may contribute a verse.
The powerful play goes on and you may contribute a verse.
What will your verse be?

What will your verse be?

Julian Wise's verse was a memorable one: "I resolved that I was going to become a lifesaver and that never again would I watch a man die when he could have been saved if those around him knew how."

That verse became his life's work.

José Rolando Aleman Brito, a twenty-three-year-old Red Cross volunteer on Isla Mujeres, writes: "I volunteered as I saw the suffering of so many people. I feel my life is worthwhile when I help others. I plan to continue helping as an ambulance driver and rescue person as long as I have the strength to do it."

Nineteen-year-old Carlos David Bacab Garrido, also from Isla Mujeres, writes: "I want to help people who have accidents and are in need."

Twice a year, cargo planes carry medical and school supplies to Isla Mujeres. Kathy Price made that happen. That is her verse. She and Judith Fernendez are now helping the people of Guatemala. That is their verse. Kathy's health continues to improve, and Judith's limp is less severe.

Kathy once said to me, "All we have are moments."

Make the most of each one.

The powerful play goes on, and you may contribute a verse.

In early January, four days after Mary Kay's funeral, Cathy and I went to Lightfoot Elementary School so we could talk to Mary Kay's sixth-grade class.

"I'm worried about them," Cathy told me. "I don't want them to be afraid."

We sat in the classroom surrounded by twelve-year-olds, and Cathy told them about what had happened to Mary Kay and then she answered all their questions.

"Mary Kay didn't have something that you could catch from her," she told them. "You can't catch what she had."

"Did she hurt?" one child asked.

"No," Cathy told him. "She didn't hurt."

More and more asked questions, and Cathy answered them all. She had been right. The children were frightened. They, too, were grieving.

"She was my friend and I'm going to miss her," came a voice from the back of the room.

"She loved all of you," Cathy told them. "You were her friends."

Cathy's verse filled the room. It eased the pain there and gave hope to children who'd lost more than a good friend. They'd lost a part of their own childhood when May Kay died.

Cathy's verse was one of love and hope.

Ten days later, Cathy and Mike and Cecelia, and young Mike and ten-year-old Anthony, were invited to attend a special memorial for Mary Kay at Lightfoot. There, friends and teachers shared remembrances of Mary Kay, and, in her memory, they planted a holly tree.

Their verse was one of love and consolation.

Jimmy Graham's verse came late one night as he was dispatching.

"I was in the middle of a bad wreck," he told me, "trying to get that dispatched and get all the units en route and the emergency phone rang again."

A two-week-old baby had stopped breathing, and the young parents didn't know what to do. Jimmy talked them through CPR, "just like on Rescue 911," he said, proudly.

The powerful play goes on.

Arthur Ashe was forty-nine years old when he died.

Arthur Ashe said he didn't just want to be remembered for playing tennis. "That's no accomplishment," he said. "That was just for me." He certainly will get his wish. He will be remembered for his goodness, the strength of his convictions, his dedication to helping young people, black and white, achieve the rights they so richly deserve.

Such was the verse of Arthur Ashe.

In October of 1992 I went to see the AIDS quilt on the Mall in Washington, D.C.

Fifteen acres, 21,000 panels: men, women, and children who have died of AIDS.

I thought that I would be overwhelmed by the magnitude of it. I was anxious about taking those last steps past the Washington Monument, stepping over the crest of the hill there . . . and facing the sea of fabric.

But it is not the immensity of it that breaks the heart.
It is the individuality of each panel . . . each one, a life.
And the farewells:
"Dad, I saw your panel. I'm still crying."
"I want to stop what could stop my generation."
"It's okay to cry."
"God doesn't make junk. He loves all."
"No more pain now. No more fears. You're at peace now."
More than 140,000 people were there to see the quilt; to mourn, to learn, and to create verses of healing.

The powerful play goes on.
David's verse comes to me from Ecuador.

People need so very little, after all,
And a fall dusk never feels commonplace,
Something to savor like a half-empty sky
Or a smooth rock found in a special place,
The sanctity of a red sun sinking into memory
Cannot be overemphasized here,
And neither can the push and pull
Of autumn winds on a dandelion puff,
A perfect, spiny sphere of
Fragile compassion.

The powerful play goes on . . .
And the verses.

This is the last chapter.
In closing, there are still things I want to say.

I want to thank you rescue volunteers for being a part of my life, for writing to me and sharing your stories with me.

I want you to be careful of "politics." Don't let egos get too big, or territories get too important. That overshadows the task at hand, which is saving lives.

Touch your patients more. For that matter, touch everyone more. If you're just getting started, the forearm is a safe place to rest your hand. If you need some encouragement, read Bernie Siegel's *Love, Medicine and Miracles*.

To get warmed up, gather your whole crew together and have a "hugment."

Talk more.
Listen better.
Be careful.
Beware of stress.
Don't be too hard on yourself! That's a tough one.
Mara's husband, Les, has told her that when she has a bad call — you know, one of those where everything goes wrong — the patient is probably fine, but your oxygen bottle was empty or you got confused over the directions or you couldn't find your scissors, or any one of a hundred things — that Mara can't make any major decision on taking some time off, quitting, etc., until she's run three good calls.

She's still going strong.

When your patient dies, try to remember that your being there gave them a chance. It's just that sometimes people can't be saved.

The powerful play goes on and you may contribute a verse.
It doesn't have to rhyme.
It just has to make a difference.

You contribute your verse each time you respond to another's needs. Your verse is in your skills and in your caring.

As the light from a star continues to shine even after the star itself has faded from the heavens, so your own special verse always will be.

God be with you.
Always.

Biography

Pat Ivey

I am still in EMS, still a cardiac technician on Lake of the Woods Volunteer Rescue Squad here in Wilderness, VA. I continue to teach EMS classes, and now I am working in the Culpeper Regional Hospital Emergency Room. I remain a great believer in holistic medicine, the magic of touch and the healing power of love. My life, as with everyone, has been a series of mountains and valleys. Since I first met Richard in 1990, I have lost my father and my older son. Both events are works in progress. The mountain in my life is my granddaughter, born in April of 2001. I've never been so in love.

Gloucester Library
P.O. Box 2380
Gloucester, VA 23061

Printed in the United States
87616LV00004B/235/A